Clinics in Human Lactation

Supplementation of the Breastfed Infant

Criteria, Decisions, and Interventions

By Marsha Walker, RN, IBCLC

Supplementation of the Breastfed Infant: Criteria, Decisions, and Interventions

Praeclarus Press, LLC
2504 Sweetgum Lane
Amarillo, Texas 79124 USA
806-367-9950
www.PraeclarusPress.com

DISCLAIMER
The information contained in this publication is advisory only and is not intended to replace sound clinical judgment or individualized patient care. The author disclaims all warranties, whether expressed or implied, including any warranty as the quality, accuracy, safety, or suitability of this information for any particular purpose.

ISBN: 978-1-939807-65-6

Table of Contents

Chapter 1. Introduction

Supplementing or complementing the breastfed infant with other fluids or foods at birth and during the early days can be traced back to ancient times. Medical opinions from as early as the Graeco-Roman period (~117 AD) recommended honey or goat's milk as the first feeding. In the 1400s, gruel was given to infants following each breastfeeding (Fildes, 1986). The early 1900s saw physicians recommending artificial foods from the first day of life to prevent the initial weight loss seen in newborns (Apple, 1987). Many physicians advised supplementing with infant formula until copious milk production was seen. Mixed feeding became more popular at the end of the 19th century and into the early 20th century, with physicians recommending supplementary bottles of infant formula to "enhance a woman's ability to lactate." It was thought that the mothers would be freed from the "duties" of breastfeeding to exercise and engage in recreation, which would help them relax and produce more milk. Even if a mother's milk supply was adequate, under the guise of "scientific motherhood" women were advised to give their infant at least one bottle a day so the mother had a little "freedom" and to make weaning easier. By the 1930s, hospital practices showed the routine use of supplemental bottles of formula for breastfed infants, as well as the distribution of prepared formula bottles upon discharge. When infants were brought to the mother to breastfeed (no such thing as rooming-in), a bottle of formula accompanied the infant. What was modeled in the hospital was repeated at home. Restrictive recommendations regarding breastfeeding, plus the supplementary bottles assured that most women would have difficulty in establishing exclusive breastfeeding. Magazine articles and advertisements extolled the virtues of infant formula and bottle-feeding, with mothers being warned to expect to use a bottle some time during infancy, even if they were already breastfeeding or planning to do so. Childcare literature through the 20th century expressed growing acceptance and the assumption that infants would be artificially fed, either partially or totally.

The most common reason mothers in the early 20th century turned to artificial feedings was the complaint of insufficient milk. This perception turned into reality when feedings were limited by strict feeding schedules promulgated by health officials, hospitals, and physicians, while magazine advertisements, friends, and family pressured mothers into formula use. Few mothers or healthcare providers recognized the actual source of the problem (Wolf, 2001). Commercial infant foods became available in the United States soon after the Civil War, were extensively advertised and easily available. As cow's milk became safer, breastfeeding fell out of favor, and by 1972 only 22 percent of newborns left the hospital breastfeeding. Further impeding breastfeeding efforts were the aggressive marketing techniques used by infant formula companies. Some physicians collaborated with infant formula companies to have instructions removed from infant formula cans and available only through physicians. Sales calls by formula detail salespeople to physicians proliferated. Free samples of infant formulas were offered by mail to readers of women's middle-class magazines. Free handbooks from formula manufacturers on infant care were offered to middle-class mothers, lending the aura of science to the artificial milk products and convincing mothers of the efficacy of feeding infant formula to their babies (Levenstein, 2003). Infant formula marketing moved into the hospital with brand name products being presented to new mothers in classes, on crib cards, and as feedings. Non-evidence-based maternity care practices ended in bottles of formula being fed by nurses to infants who seldom saw their mothers during the many days of her hospital stay. Both mothers and physicians started doubting the ability of most women to breastfeed. Breastfeeding experienced a resurgence when La Leche League was formed in 1956 and in the 1970s when natural childbirth and family centered birthing rooms paved the way for an increase in breastfeeding rates. While breastfeeding initiation rates increased, many of these infants were still supplemented with formula in the hospital. Exclusive breastfeeding rates remained low and fluctuated over time (Table 1.1).

Table 1.1. Formula Supplementation Trends in the Hospital

1971
21% exclusively breastfeeding in hospital
Additional 3% supplemented with infant formula
1982
55% exclusively breastfeeding in hospital
Additional 6.9% supplemented with infant formula
2001
46.3% exclusively breastfeeding in hospital
Additional 23% supplemented with infant formula
2003
44% exclusively breastfeeding in hospital
Additional 22% supplemented with infant formula
2006
38.4% exclusively breastfeeding in hospital
Additional 25.2% supplemented with infant formula

Source: Ryan, A.S., Wenjun, Z., & Acosta, A. (2002). Breastfeeding continues to increase into the new millennium. *Pediatrics, 110,* 1103-1109; Mothers Survey, Ross Products, Breastfeeding Trends—2003, 2006.

The Extent and Effect of the Problem

The ingrained intervention of formula supplementation persists into the 21st century, often started during the hospital stay following childbirth and continued or begun after discharge home. Mothers who supplement with formula in the hospital or during the early postpartum period rarely return to exclusive breastfeeding (Sarasua, Clausen, & Frunchak, 2009; Hill, Humenick, Brennan, & Woolley, 1997). The 2013 *Breastfeeding Report Card* from the Centers for Disease Control and Prevention (CDC) showed that even though nationally 76.5% of infants have ever been breastfed, nearly a quarter of them receive formula supplementation before two days of age.[1] In some states up to 35% of newborns receive formula supplementation prior to two days of age. Most mothers who wish to exclusively breastfeed intend to do so for longer than three months, but the majority of these mothers are not meeting their intended goal. Mothers are more likely to achieve their intended breastfeeding goal when formula supplementation is avoided in the hospital. Numerous studies illustrate the pervasiveness and extent of non-evidence-based formula supplementation in the hospital:

- In a study by Perrine, Scanlon, Li, Odom, and Grummer-Strawn (2012), 40% of the 1,457 infants studied received supplemental formula feedings in the hospital in spite of maternal intensions to exclusively breastfeed. There was a substantial gap between exclusive breastfeeding intention and exclusive breastfeeding duration. Only 32.4% of women surveyed achieved their exclusive breastfeeding intention, a disappointing statistic for both mothers and public health.

- In a sample of 726 mothers, Kurinij and Shiono (1991) reported that 37% of breastfed infants were given formula supplementation in the hospital. A concerning finding was that 50% of the infants whose mothers delivered at a public or community hospital were supplemented, compared with 15% of the newborns delivered at a university hospital. Women giving birth where the supplementation rates were lowest were 3.5 times more likely to be exclusively breastfeeding. The longer a mother waited to initiate breastfeeding, the more likely she was to use formula, illustrating the importance of facilitating breastfeeding within an hour or so of birth. Seventeen reasons were cited for supplementing breastfed infants, with the top three being (1) to give the mother some rest, (2) because the mother was ill, or (3) because the mother did not have enough breastmilk.

---

1 http://www.cdc.gov/breastfeeding/pdf/2013BreastfeedingReportCard.pdf

- Tender et al. (2009) reported that of 150 low-income mothers, 60% initiated breastfeeding and 78% of these breastfed infants received formula supplementation while hospitalized. Only 13% of these infants received supplementation according to the evidence-based supplementation guidelines from the Academy of Breastfeeding Medicine (2009). Reasons for supplementation included the mother's perception of not enough milk and that her milk was not in at birth. Providers' reasons for supplementation included that the infant was lactose intolerant, it was necessary to help simplify weaning, the mother was taking medications, and to allow the mother to sleep. Over 20% of mothers did not know why their infant was supplemented. Within the cohort of women receiving WIC benefits, 80% of breastfed infants were given supplements in the hospital, 87% of which was medically unnecessary. Infants of mothers who did not attend a prenatal breastfeeding class were 4.7 times more likely to receive formula supplementation in hospital. This study demonstrated the importance of improving medical providers' knowledge about breastfeeding and medical indications for supplementation, as well as the necessity of correcting misinformation on the part of the mother.

- Crivelli-Kovach and Chung (2011) described current breastfeeding policies and practices among Philadelphia hospitals and changes in their policies and practices over time. Of the 18 participating hospitals, 40% of them reported that breastfed infants were receiving formula supplementation over 50% of the time, and 68% reported that supplements were given at the mother's request. Most hospitals (89%) reported giving formula supplements compared with 37% in 1994 and 1999. The increased use of formula supplements over time indicates the need for specific supplementation policies in hospitals.

- Biro, Sutherland, Yelland, Hardy, and Brown (2011) reported that 23% of the 4,085 women who initiated breastfeeding in their study had infants who were supplemented with formula. Infants were more likely to be supplemented if the mother was primiparous (perhaps indicating a lack of confidence and/or knowledge), if the mother had a body mass index (BMI) of more than 30 (obesity can delay lactogenesis II), if the mother had a cesarean section (cesareans can delay the time to first breastfeed and the onset of copious milk production), if the infant was low birth weight or admitted to the special care nursery (separation and rush to feed formula), or if the infant was born in a hospital without the Baby

Friendly Hospital Initiative (BFHI) designation (indicating a higher risk of non-evidence-based practices). Primiparous mothers were twice as likely to provide formula supplementation to their infant. First-time mothers may lack knowledge of the early breastfeeding process and be anxious regarding their ability to satisfy the infant's hunger. This was seen in a study by Semenic, Loiselle & Gottlieb (2008) who found that in-hospital formula supplementation by first-time mothers was associated with perceived breastfeeding problems and lower breastfeeding self-efficacy.

• Gagnon, Leduc, Waghorn, Yang, and Platt (2005) analyzed 564 breastfeeding mother/infant pairs to understand reasons for in-hospital supplementation. Almost half of the infants (47.9%) received formula in the hospital. The researchers also discovered that the highest risk time of day for an infant to receive supplementation was between 7:00 p.m. and 9:00 a.m., regardless of the time of birth. Nurses in this study revealed that "insufficient milk" was a common reason for supplementing, even though it is rare for a mother to have true "milk insufficiency" at this point in time. Infant behaviors, such as fussiness, sleepiness, or latching difficulties, often triggered supplementation, even though there are numerous breastfeeding interventions that can address these issues and do not involve formula supplementation. Highly anxious mothers were a subgroup of women who needed extra support and special interventions to avoid unnecessary supplementation. High maternal trait anxiety resulted in 2.5 times more supplementation in the hospital.

• In a population of low-income women, Bolton, Chow, Benton, and Olson (2009) reported that formula introduction on day one postpartum was associated with a significantly shorter breastfeeding duration and that the most dramatic predictor of a shorter breastfeeding duration was introduction of formula on day one. In this study formula supplementation on day one resulted in a 38- to 49-day shorter length of breastfeeding duration. Since early weaning is associated with the early introduction of formula (Hornell, Hofvander, & Kylberg, 2001), delaying formula introduction may be highly effective in lengthening the duration of exclusive breastfeeding.

• Latina or Hispanic women initiate breastfeeding at fairly high rates, but their exclusive breastfeeding rates are much lower. In a study by Newton, Chaudhuri, Grossman, and Merewood

(2009) of 325 Hispanic mothers who initiated breastfeeding, 229 mothers supplemented with four or more formula feeds, but in 79% of these cases, no reason was recorded in the medical record for formula supplementation. The mean time to the first formula feeding was 14.6 hours, a disappointing start to the breastfeeding experience.

- Hall et al. (2002) found that babies given two or more bottles of formula within the first 24 hours demonstrated a significant risk for breastfeeding cessation at 7-10 days.

- Even just one bottle of formula can affect the duration of breastfeeding. Chezem, Friesen, Montgomery, Fortman, and Clark (1998) looked at the patterns of human milk replacement during hospitalization. In a small sample of 53 mothers, 28% of the infants received at least one formula bottle while in the hospital. The duration of breastfeeding was significantly shorter in women whose infants received any formula during hospitalization (nine weeks) compared with women whose infants were not fed formula (20 weeks). Only 40% of the infants fed formula in the hospital were still breastfeeding at six weeks compared with 88% of those not fed formula.

- Use of daily human milk replacements is negatively correlated with breastfeeding duration, regardless of the mother's prenatal intentions to exclusively or partially breastfeed (Chezem, Friesen, & Boettcher, 2003). The provision of formula bottles can be the cause of breastfeeding problems or a symptom of breastfeeding difficulties. Infants who are given non-breastmilk fluids in the first 48 hours, or offered pacifiers, have been shown to be two to three times more likely to have suboptimal breastfeeding behaviors on days three and seven (Infant Breastfeeding Assessment Tool score < 10), interfering with the establishment of effective breastfeeding (Dewey, Nommsen-Rivers, Heinig, & Cohen, 2003).

- Sievers, Haase, Oldigs, and Schaub (2003) studied peripartum indicators in mothers and infants who were most at risk for early lactation failure. Partial feeding of infant formula or an intake of less than 150 g (5.3 oz) of human milk per day 24-48 hours after lactogenesis II was linked to weaning within four weeks.

- Over 40 years of research has shown that the introduction of breastmilk substitutes (water or formula), whether in the hospital or in the first month of life, has a consistently negative effect on breastfeeding duration. Blomquist, Jonsbo, Serenius and Persson (1994) found that breastfed infants who had been given supplements in the hospital were almost four times more likely to have weaned by three months of age and were seven times less likely to be breastfed at three months if they experienced in-hospital supplementation and experienced a loss of 10% birth weight or more. However, among infants receiving supplements for the specific indications of maternal insulin-dependent diabetes mellitus or gestational diabetes, the duration of breastfeeding was similar to that in the non-supplemented group. Supplementation without a medical reason significantly reduces the duration of both exclusive and partial breastfeeding; conversely, supplementation for medical reasons did not have this type of dramatic effect on intensity or duration of breastfeeding in this study (Ekstrom, Widstrom, & Nissen, 2003).

- Unnecessary supplementation has a marked effect on lactogenesis III, or the calibration and maintenance of a sufficient milk supply (Daly, Owens, & Hartmann, 1993). This is especially true if there is no care plan or if the mother is not instructed to express her milk on a regular basis during the time that supplementation is being given. This interference with the body's ability to accomplish and sustain copious milk production can result in reduced amounts of breastmilk transferred to the infant (Drewett et al., 1989) and a repeating cycle of more formula supplementation until the body receives the signal for breast involution. Breastfeeding frequency and duration decline quickly after the start of regular formula supplementation (one or more bottles of formula per day). The younger the age of the infant when started on regular formula supplementation, the sooner breastfeeding will be abandoned (Hornell, Hofvander, & Kylberg, 2001). The most frequent reason for supplementing young infants is the mother's impression that she does not have enough milk to satisfy the infant. Whether this shortage is real or merely perceived, intervention is needed to prevent the downward spiral toward weaning.

- Breastfeeding intensity or degree of exclusivity has been shown to be predictive of duration of breastfeeding up to one year of age. Petrova, Hegyi, and Mehta (2007) found that women who exclusively breastfed in the hospital were more likely to be exclusively breastfeeding at one month compared with mothers who introduced formula during the hospital stay. Among mothers exclusively breastfeeding in the hospital, 50.9% were exclusively breastfeeding at the end of the first month, compared with 20.3% of mothers who introduced formula during their hospital stay. Hill, Humenick, Brennan, and Woolley (1997) followed 343 mothers for 20 weeks or until weaning, observing the supplementation patterns and subsequent rate of breastfeeding at five months postpartum. The breastfeeding rate at 20 weeks was significantly greater for mothers who reported feeding breastmilk exclusively at two weeks postpartum (~61%) compared with mothers who supplemented with formula (~26%). The strongest association with breastfeeding duration of one year has been shown to be higher breastfeeding intensity during months four through six postpartum (Piper & Parks, 2001).

- Hispanic infants are at a high risk for being supplemented with not only formula, but also tea and water. Wojcicki et al. (2011) reported that of 192 Latina mothers in their study, 44.7% of the breastfed infants were supplemented with formula by four to six weeks, 9% were fed breastmilk with water or tea, and 37.4% were exclusively breastfed. Including the exclusively formula-fed infants, 25.4% of all of the infants in this study were supplemented with water or tea at four to six weeks. Supplementing breastfed infants with water and/or tea increases the risk of micronutrient deficiencies from a diet of reduced breastmilk.

- The Listening to Mothers III study conducted by the Childbirth Connection surveyed 2,400 mothers regarding their experiences with childbirth and the immediate postpartum period who had delivered their infant during the period from July 1, 2011 through June 30, 2012 (Declercq, Sakala, Corry, Applebaum, & Herrlich, 2013). As women neared the end of their pregnancies, 54% reported wanting to breastfeed exclusively, while 27% planned to use a combination of breastfeeding and formula, and 19% planned to use formula only. One week after giving birth, half (50%) of the mothers reported feeding their babies breastmilk only. Among mothers who had given birth at least seven months earlier, 29% reported exclusive breastfeeding for at least six months. Of those mothers who intended to exclusively breastfeed, 49% were given free formula samples or offers, 37% of their babies were given pacifiers by staff, and about three in ten (29%) were given formula or water to supplement their breastmilk during the hospital stay. Most major health organizations and agencies recommend exclusive breastfeeding for the first six months followed by the addition of appropriate complementary foods, with breastfeeding continuing to a year or more (Table 1.2). Contrary to these guidelines and recommendations, in a follow-up of survey participants[2] who intended to exclusively breastfeed, the following was reported:

- 49% were given free formula samples or offers

- 47% were not told about breastfeeding resources in their communities

- 37% of their babies were given pacifiers by staff

- 36% were not shown how to position the baby to limit nipple soreness

- 35% of babies did not "room in" with their mothers while in the hospital

- 31% were not encouraged to breastfeed on demand

- 29% were given formula or water to supplement their mother's breastmilk

- 19% did not receive help to start breastfeeding when they were ready

The survey also found that both their intention to exclusively breastfeed and actually doing so a week after the birth fell substantially as the number of prior children increased.

---

2   http://transform.childbirthconnection.org/reports/listeningtomothers/breastfeeding/

Table 1.2. Health Organizations and Agencies Recommending Exclusive Breastfeeding for the First Six Months

American Academy of Family Physicians (2008)
Academy of Nutrition and Dietetics (formerly American Dietetic Association) (2009)
American Academy of Pediatrics (2012)
American Congress of Obstetricians and Gynecologists (formerly American College of Obstetricians and Gynecologists) (2007)
American College of Nurse Midwives (2011)
American Public Health Association (2007)
Centers for Disease Control and Prevention (2013a)

The U.S. Department of Health and Human Services (HHS) has promulgated breastfeeding goals for the nation for three decades through the Healthy People initiative. The initiative provides science-based, 10-year national objectives for improving the health of all Americans. Among the breastfeeding objectives for 2020 is included the improvement of exclusive breastfeeding rates to 46.2% at three months and 25.5% at six months.[3] Reaching these goals represents an ambitious investment in maternal and infant health, as supplementation can be a complex issue. Numerous factors are associated with supplementation of breastfed infants (Table 1.3). Some factors are non-modifiable and require increased surveillance and more intense provision of maternal and provider education and interventions. Other factors can be modified to create a more conducive environment for exclusive breastfeeding.

Table 1.3. Factors Associated With Supplementation of Breastfed Infants

Factors	Reference
Low birth weight, African American, smoking in the home, mothers less than 20 years of age, mothers with poor mental or emotional health	Jones, Kogan, Singh, Dee, & Grummer Strawn (2011)
Not being breastfed within one hour of birth	DiFrisco, Goodman, Budin, Lilienthal, Kleinman, & Holmes (2011)
Score of less than 6.9 on LATCH assessment, cesarean section, primiparity, infant phototherapy	Tornese, Ronfani, Pavan, Demarini, Monasta, & Davanzo (2012)

---

3 http://www.healthypeople.gov/2020/topicsobjectives2020/objectiveslist.aspx?topicId=26

Maternal request due to inadequate knowledge of newborn behaviors and feeding capabilities, lack of understanding of breastfeeding physiology, formula as a solution for breastfeeding problems, fussy baby	DaMota, Banuelos, Goldbronn, Vera-Beccera, & Heinig (2012)
Problems with infant latching on or sucking, healthcare provider recommendation of formula	Taveras, Li, Grummer-Strawn, Richardson, Marshall, Rego, Miroshnik, & Lieu (2004)
Pacifier restriction without also restricting formula supplementation, lack of provision of information on infant soothing techniques	Kair, Kenron, Etheredge, Jaffe, & Phillipi (2013)
Lack of an evidence-based breastfeeding protocol in pediatric office practices	Corriveau, Drake, Kellams, & Rovnyak (2013)
Mother's perception of insufficient milk or milk had not come in at birth, lack of attendance at prenatal breastfeeding class, lack of evidence-based healthcare provider knowledge	Tender, Janakiram, Arce, Mason, Jordan, Marsh, Kin, He, & Moon (2009)
Primiparous, body mass index more than 30, cesarean, baby admitted to special care, baby born in hospital without Baby Friendly designation	Biro, Sutherland, Yelland, Hardy, & Brown (2011)
So someone else can feed the baby, so the infant does not experience hunger, so the baby is full, so the baby will not cry with hunger, so the baby is healthy, so the mother can be employed, Hispanic mother	Waldrop (2013)
Baby wasn't getting enough, not sucking long enough, latch difficulties, difficulty accessing lactation consultants, minimal efforts to breastfeed, formula bottles in the hospital, reluctance to call for help post discharge, return to work	Cottrell & Detman (2013)

Where a mother delivers can have a profound effect on the exclusivity of breastfeeding. Rates of exclusive breastfeeding vary widely from hospital to hospital. For example, exclusive breastfeeding rates in California hospitals range from a low of 8.6% to a high of 95.4%.[4] Hospitals with the Baby Friendly designation tend to have breastfeeding rates above both national and regional levels (Merewood, Mehta, Chamberlain, Philipp, & Bauchner, 2005). Abrahams and Labbok (2009) found that implementation of the international BFHI was associated with a statistically significant annual increase in rates of exclusive breastfeeding among infants zero to two months of age and among infants zero to six months of age in the 14 countries studied.

The CDC recognized the high rates of formula supplementation and the resultant low rates of exclusive breastfeeding as a public health issue and started monitoring in-hospital formula supplementation rates and other hospital maternity care practices through a national survey entitled Maternity Practices in Infant Nutrition and Care (mPINC).[5] The mPINC survey began in 2007 and is administered every two years to all birthing centers and hospitals with a maternal/newborn service. Results of mPINC surveys from 2007, 2009, and 2011 showed that less than a quarter of the surveyed hospitals limited the use of infant formula, water, or glucose supplements for healthy full-term infants (Perrine, Shealy, Scanlon, Grummer-Strawn, & Galuska, 2011; Centers for Disease Control and Prevention, 2013b). According to the 2011 mPINC survey, 18% of facilities give breastfed infants glucose water and 23.7% of facilities supplement between 50-89% of breastfed newborns.

This troubling trend was also recognized by the Joint Commission, the organization that accredits and certifies hospitals. Starting in 2014, the Joint Commission will require that hospitals with 1,100 or more births per year report on the Perinatal Care Core Measure set, which includes collection of data on exclusive breastmilk feeding.[6] Exclusive breastmilk feeding will be a performance measure requirement, with the Joint Commission wanting to see an increase in the rate of exclusive breastmilk feeding over time. The Joint Commission realizes that implementation of evidence-based best practices for infant feeding, such as those recommended in the Baby Friendly Hospital Initiative,[7] will reduce the number of infants who receive formula supplementation for non-medical reasons and increase the number of exclusively breastmilk-fed infants at discharge. The Joint Commission makes the distinction between exclusive breastfeeding and exclusive breastmilk feeding. This distinction allows infants with breastfeeding difficulties to be supplemented with human milk and still be

4   http://cdm16254.contentdm.oclc.org/cdm/singleitem/collection/p178601ccp2/id/1179/rec/8

5   http://www.cdc.gov/breastfeeding/data/mpinc/index.htm

6   https://manual.jointcommission.org/releases/TJC2013A/MIF0170.html

7   http://www.babyfriendlyusa.org/

counted as exclusively breastmilk fed. Even with exemplary lactation care and services, the Joint Commission realizes that in any hospital there will always be a small number of breastfed infants who require supplementation due to medical indications. There may also be maternal circumstances which necessitate that supplementation be implemented until the mother is able to directly breastfeed the infant or express sufficient milk. The CDC's mPINC survey suggests that fewer than 10% of breastfed infants should receive supplemental formula in the hospital. This can be used as a benchmark in hospitals working to reduce the number of breastfed infants who are supplemented with formula.

As part of attaining the BFHI designation as a Baby Friendly hospital, Step 6 criteria states that hospitals are to supplement breastfed infants when there is a medical indication—not routinely, not for convenience, not necessarily with formula, and not as the first line intervention for early breastfeeding difficulties. Hospitals working towards the Baby Friendly designation follow the Ten Steps to Successful Breastfeeding (Table 1.4). The *Ten Steps to Successful Breastfeeding* were developed by a team of global experts and consist of evidence-based practices that have been shown to increase breastfeeding initiation, duration, and exclusivity. Baby Friendly hospitals and birthing facilities must adhere to the Ten Steps to receive and retain a Baby Friendly designation. A year-by-year reduction in non-medically indicated supplementation is expected in Baby Friendly designated facilities.

One way hospitals have helped restrict supplemental formula use in breastfed infants to actual medical indications is to lock up the formula and require staff to log out the formula, noting the formula batch number in case there is a recall, date and time of formula use, patient and staff members' names, and reason for use. Some hospitals manage formula use by placing it in a medication distribution system such as Pyxis. This helps provide information on where additional staff education may be needed and helps reduce unnecessary formula supplementation (Cadwell & Turner-Maffei, 2009).

Table 1.4. Ten Steps to Successful Breastfeeding

1. Have a written breastfeeding policy that is routinely communicated to all health care staff.

2. Train all health care staff in the skills necessary to implement this policy.

3. Inform all pregnant women about the benefits and management of breastfeeding.

4. Help mothers initiate breastfeeding within one hour of birth.

5. Show mothers how to breastfeed and how to maintain lactation, even if they are separated from their infants.

6. Give infants no food or drink other than breast milk, unless medically indicated.

7. Practice rooming in—allow mothers and infants to remain together 24 hours a day.

8. Encourage breastfeeding on demand.

9. Give no pacifiers or artificial nipples to breastfeeding infants.

10. Foster the establishment of breastfeeding support groups and refer mothers to them on discharge from the hospital or birth center.

Source: World Health Organization: *Protecting, promoting and supporting breast-feeding: the special role of maternity services.* Geneva: World Health Organization; 1989.

Commercial Pressure to Supplement with Infant Formula

Commercial pressure to supplement breastfeeding with formula capitalizes on new mothers' insecurities and concerns over breastfeeding adequacy, and is fed by healthcare provider endorsement of the practice and unrelenting advertising by formula manufacturers. Distributing formula company discharge bags to new mothers when they leave the hospital is another form of supplementation with commercial overtones. These bags represent a marketing tactic (not a gift) designed to cause breastfeeding mothers to supplement with formula and purchase more of the product, thus creating a market where none existed before (Walker, 2007). HIPAA defines this practice as a form of marketing.[8] HIPAA does not require authorization from the mother stating that she understands that this "gift" is actually part of a formula marketing scheme. Women who received these commercial bags were more likely to exclusively breastfeed for fewer than ten weeks than were women who had not received the formula company

---

8   http://www.hhs.gov/ocr/privacy/hipaa/understanding/coveredentities/marketing.pdf

bags (Rosenberg, Eastham, & Kasehagen, 2008). The distribution of these bags to new mothers by hospitals is part of a long-standing marketing campaign by infant formula manufacturers and implies hospital and staff endorsement of infant formula. This practice presents a mixed message to new mothers, with hospitals and staff acting as a marketing conduit for formula manufacturers. Many hospitals have recognized the ethical problems created by commercial relationships with infant formula manufacturers and have eliminated the distribution of formula company bags. They have created their own bags, marketing their birthing services rather than allowing formula company access to their patients. Over 800 U.S. hospitals have eliminated these bags, often with help from the Ban the Bags campaign (www.banthebags.org), which provides materials and assistance with formula company bag elimination.

While the American Academy of Pediatrics (AAP) supports and encourages breastfeeding (American Academy of Pediatrics, 2012), it still seems to condone and promote the practice of formula supplementation through commercial formula bag distribution (Figure 1.1).

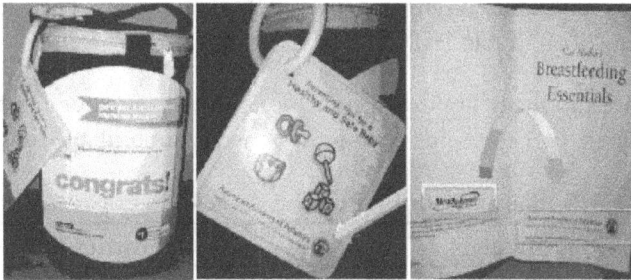

Figure 1.1. AAP materials on formula discharge bag
Source: Courtesy MotherBaby Summit. Used with permission.

AAP materials appear on and in a commercial formula discharge bag. This presents a contradicting and confusing situation for both mothers and clinicians. It is difficult to reconcile AAP breastfeeding recommendations with such a practice. This gives the appearance that breastfeeding mothers will need to use formula, that this is normal, and that the AAP endorses formula supplementation using this particular brand.

Commercial pressure to supplement with formula intensified when manufacturers introduced formula specifically labeled for breastfeeding supplementation. One manufacturer's website normalizes formula supplementation by stating that, "8 out of 10 moms who supplemented with formula agreed that it helped them to continue to feed breastmilk."[9] Clicking on the formula icon takes mothers to a page that states, "You

---

9   https://similac.com/baby-formula/similac-for-supplementation

might notice several differences in how your baby eats after you begin supplementing breastmilk with formula. If your baby refuses the breast, eats faster, goes longer than usual between feedings, or does not pass stool after a few days, don't be overly concerned—these changes are common and do not always signal a problem. If these conditions last longer than a few days, or if you have questions about your baby's health, contact your pediatrician about possible milk intolerance."[10] Breast refusal for a few days can provoke an end to breastfeeding and poses potential harm for both mother and baby. The negative outcomes of this practice are glossed over or not even mentioned.

At the same time that these supplementing formulas were introduced, an article appeared in the journal *Pediatrics*, a publication of the American Academy of Pediatrics, which concluded that early formula supplementation would improve breastfeeding duration and that restricting formula supplementation during the birth hospitalization could be detrimental for some subpopulations of healthy-term newborns (Flaherman, Aby, et al., 2013). As the conclusions of this article are controversial, a number of criticisms and shortcomings of the methodology have been identified[11] (Furman, 2013) (Table 1.5).

There are too many important limitations to this study design that cause questioning of the conclusion and the generalization of the results.

Table 1.5. Problems With Flaherman Article

Concerns	Comments
Small sample size	20 breastfed infants; 20 formula-supplemented infants
Enrolled infants at 5% below birth weight at ≤ 36 hours of age	Evidence does not consider such infants to be at risk
Used infant formula for supplementation	Why wasn't expressed colostrum or donor human milk used for supplementation

10 http://similac.com/feeding-nutrition/supplementing/formula-supplementing
11 http://bfmed.wordpress.com/2013/05/13/early-limited-data-for-early-limited-formula-use/

Mothers had to agree that they did not mind their infant receiving infant formula	Mothers were not informed of potential side effects of gut microbiome alteration, reduced milk supply with no expressing
Amount of formula supplemented was almost the same as the total volume of colostrum a newborn would normally consume	Could serve to reduce colostrum intake and number of breastfeeds per 24 hours
Weight loss calculations did not account for diuresis and meconium stooling	Both diuresis of excess fluid and large meconium stooling can cause early infant weight loss, neither of which are indicative of feeding difficulties or signal the necessity for supplementation
Misleading headlines stating that syringe-feeding breastfed newborns 10 ml of formula after every breastfeeding will prolong breastfeeding duration	Misinterpretation by hospital clinicians that infant formula supplementation is benign, normal, and necessary
Descriptions were lacking regarding the guidelines mothers were given for breastfeeding their infants	Poor lactation assessment and/or support, lack of documentation of swallowing, absence of guidance for preventing excessive weight loss could have contributed to infant weight loss
One of the authors of the article serves as a consultant for four formula companies	This could bias both the reason for the study and the outcomes

Chapter 2. Why Just Breastmilk? Effect of Formula on the Microbiome of the Breastfed Infant's Gut

While there are certainly negative ramifications of non-medically indicated formula supplementation on exclusivity and duration of breastfeeding, on maternal milk production, and on health outcomes of both mothers and infants due to abbreviated periods of exclusive or any breastfeeding, there are immediate alterations in the microbiome of the newborn gut when formula is introduced. Within the human gut lives the microbiota, an enormous and diverse community of microorganisms, the bulk of which is bacteria that have a vital role in the development of intestinal functions and in the life-long health of the individual. Gut microbiota influence the growth and differentiation of the gut's epithelial cells and are central to nutritive, metabolic, immunological, and protective functions. Bacterial cells far outnumber the human cells in the gastrointestinal tract and the total amount of genes in the various bacterial species greatly exceed the number of human genes. The totality of gut microorganisms, their genetic elements, and their environmental interactions is known as the microbiome. This gut microbiome has been called an "organ within an organ" as it is capable of executing enzymatic reactions and modulating gene expression involved in mucosal barrier fortification, angiogenesis, and intestinal maturation following birth.

The gut (intestine) is the largest interface between the body and the external environment and contains 60-70 percent of the immune system. Its dual role allows absorption of nutrients while performing as a barrier to prevent pathogens, toxins, and antigens from entering the body and causing acute or chronic diseases and conditions. Illness and conditions associated with intestinal barrier dysfunction are more common in adults who were formula fed as infants compared with those who were breastfed (Verhasselt, 2010). This intestinal barrier contains four main components, the physical, chemical, immunological, and microbiological (Figure 2.1).

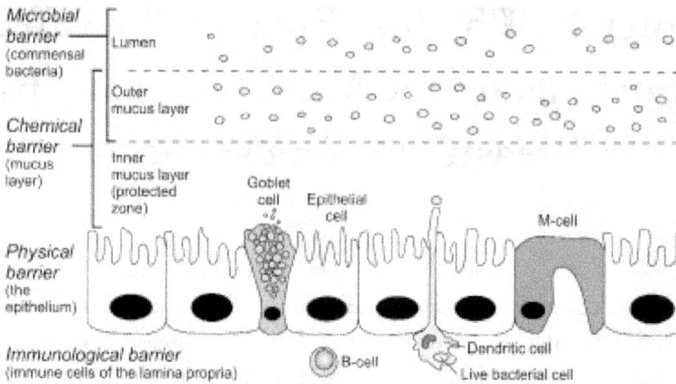

Figure 2.1. Intestinal barriers
Source: © 2012 Anderson, Dalziel, Gopal, Bassett, Ellis and Roy. Originally published in: http://dx.doi.org/10.5772/25753 under CC BY 3.0 license. Used with permission.

The physical barrier is the first line of defense and is composed of a layer of columnar epithelial cells between which are the tight junctions. The tight junctions control gut permeability, allowing passage of fluids, electrolytes, and small macromolecules, but preventing the passage of larger macromolecules. The gut is permeable during fetal life and early after birth. Gut closure or closure of the tight junctions starts during the first postnatal week. Any delay, change, or insult to the gut that changes this process predisposes the infant to infection, inflammatory states, and allergic sensitization (Maheshwari & Zemlin, 2009). The gut-closure process is mediated by hormones and growth factors in human milk that facilitate epithelial growth and maturation.

It has long been accepted that the gut of a term fetus is sterile and that the bacterial colonization of the newborn gut does not occur until after transit through the birth canal, where maternal vaginal and fecal bacteria become the first residents. However, newer research has shown that infants may develop their original gut microbiome while still in the womb. Researchers have reported that the meconium of term infants is not a sterile environment, with gut colonization starting before birth (Jimenez et al., 2008). Bacteria can be isolated from amniotic fluid without any clinical or histological evidence of infection or inflammation in either the mother or the infant. Since the fetus continuously swallows amniotic fluid in utero, bacteria present in amniotic fluid from the maternal digestive tract may be the origin of the first infant gut colonizers. This suggests that the bacterial composition of the maternal gut could affect the bacterial content seen in infant meconium and serve as the pioneer bacteria colonizing the fetal gut. A study looking at meconium microbiota in term newborns found that meconium samples clustered into two types with different bacterial diversity and composition. One type was less diverse, dominated by enteric bacteria and associated with a history of atopic eczema in the mother, and the other was dominated by lactic acid bacteria and associated with respiratory problems in the infant. The mothers' lifestyle also affected the first bacterial communities in the meconium, with mothers who consumed organic foods during pregnancy promoting the lactic acid bacteria and mothers who smoked encouraging an enteric microbiome. The authors suggested that oxidative stress might also influence which type of bacteria reaches the fetus through effects on inflammation and immune function. Organic farming decreases free radicals and increases the antioxidants present in food. Smoking, on the other hand, could increase oxidative stress as cigarette smoke contains high levels of free radicals. Organic food consumption could directly affect the type of bacteria in the mother's gastrointestinal system, as organic farming influences the bacterial communities in the soil, crops, and animals directly modifying the exposure of bacteria through the food chain. Thus, maternal immune factors, as well as maternal health and lifestyle, can all contribute to the diversity and type of bacteria that first reach the fetal gut (Gosalbes et al., 2013).

Further acquisition of the infant's gut flora occurs during and after delivery through a number of mechanisms and routes:

- Mode of delivery – during a vaginal delivery, bacteria from maternal vaginal and intestinal microbiota colonize the infant gut. During a cesarean delivery, infants are deprived of contact with the maternal vaginal microbiota and experience a deficiency of strict anaerobes, such as *E. coli, Bacteroides,* and *Bifidobacteria,* and a higher presence of facultative anaerobes, such as *Clostridium* species, compared with vaginally born infants (Adlerberth & Wold, 2009).

- Gestational age – the pattern of gut colonization in preterm infants differs from that of healthy-term infants. This deviation in colonization is due to a number of factors, including the use of sterile infant formula and antibiotics, which could also contribute to feeding intolerance and in the development of necrotizing enterocolitis (Neu & Walker, 2011). Preterm infants are also often born by cesarean section, are colonized with fewer bacteria, and are exposed to pathogenic institutional organisms.

- Feeding modality – newborns also acquire gut colonizing bacteria from their mother's milk. Breastmilk is thought to be one of the most important postpartum elements modulating the metabolic and immunologic programming relative to a child's health (Aaltonen et al., 2011). Breastmilk is not sterile, nor is it meant to be. Researchers have identified more than 700 bacterial species in human milk that vary from mother to mother depending on mode of delivery and the obesity status of the mother. Colostrum has an even higher diversity of bacterial species than transitional or mature milk (Cabrera-Rubio et al., 2012). Overweight and obesity is associated with an inflammation-prone aberrant gut microbiota which can be transferred to the infant, provoking an unfavorable metabolic development (Collado, Isolauri, Laitinen, & Salminen, 2010). An unfavorable or abnormal microbial colonization during the early weeks and months of life interferes with many functions in the gut as well as provokes a slower postnatal maturation of epithelial cell barrier functions, which alters the permeability of the gut and facilitates invasion of pathogens and foreign or harmful antigens (Perrier & Corthesy, 2011). This perinatal period is a critical time where "set points" are imprinted in the neonatal gut. The nature of the microbiota acquired during the perinatal period are crucial in determining the intestinal immune response and tolerance such that alterations of the gut environment are directly responsible for mucosal inflammation and disease, autoimmunity conditions, and allergic disorders in childhood and adulthood (Gronlund, Arvilommi, Kero, Lehtonen, & Isolauri, 2000).

The Gut Microbiome of the Breastfed and Formula-Fed Infant are Different

Breastfed and formula-fed infants demonstrate a marked and impressive difference in their respective gut microbiota (Mountzouris, McCartney, & Gibson, 2002). Compared with formula-fed infants, breastfed infants develop a lower gut pH (acidic environment) of approximately 5.1-5.4 throughout the first six weeks of life, which is dominated by Bifidobacterium, and a reduced population of pathogenic (disease-causing) microbes, such as numerous species of *Escherichia coli*, *Bacteroides*, clostridia, enterococci, and streptococci. Infants fed formula have a high gut pH of approximately 5.9-7.3 characterized by a variety of putrefactive bacterial species. In infants fed breastmilk plus formula supplements, the mean pH is approximately 5.7-6.0 during the first four weeks after birth, falling to 5.45 by the sixth week. Supplementation with formula induces a rapid shift in the gut bacterial pattern of a breastfed infant. The dominance of bifidobacterium during exclusive breastfeeding decreases when infant formula is added to the diet (Favier, Vaughan, De Vos, & Akkermans, 2002). If breastfed infants receive infant formula supplementation during the first seven days of life, the production of a strongly acidic gut environment is delayed and its full potential may never be reached. Breastfed infants who receive supplements develop gut flora and behavior like those of formula-fed infants. The probability of an infant being appropriately colonized by bifidobacterium is reduced when the mother has a high body mass index (i.e., is obese), the mother experiences excessive weight gain during pregnancy, and the baby is delivered by cesarean section. The probability of appropriate bifidobacterial colonization is higher when the mother is of normal weight, has appropriate bifidobacterial colonization in her own gut and in her breastmilk, and is actively breastfeeding (Isolauri, 2012). Another bacterial group found in breastfed infants that is almost as widespread as *Bifidobacteria* is the genus Ruminococcus (Morelli, 2008). Ruminococcus serves a protective function because it produces the bactericidal ruminococcin, which inhibits the development of many of the pathologic species of *Clostridium* (Dabard et al., 2001). One notable difference between the microbiota of breastfed and formula-fed infants is the low presence of clostridia in breastfed infants as compared with formula-fed infants. Results from the use of new molecular biology techniques have detected the presence of the genus Desulfovibrio, mainly in formula-fed infants (Hopkins, Macfarlane, Furrie, Fite, & Macfarlane, 2005; Stewart, Chadwick, & Murray, 2006). These organisms have been linked with the development of inflammatory bowel disease. Zhang, Lee, Truneh, Everett, and Parker (2012) described a unique property of human milk that fosters a certain type of growth feature of bacterial colonies in the gut of newborn breastfed infants. These researchers grew bacteria (non-pathologic *E. coli* that are normal inhabitants of the gut) in samples of infant formula, cow's milk, and breastmilk. Within minutes, the bacteria began multiplying in all of the specimens, but there was a dramatic difference in the manner in which the bacteria grew. In the breastmilk specimens, the bacteria stuck together forming biofilms - thin, adherent layers of bacteria that serve as a shield against pathogens. Bacteria in the infant formula and cow's milk specimens proliferated wildly, but grew as individual organisms that did not aggregate to form protective barriers.

Alteration of gut microbiota in infants during the early critical developmental window has been linked to a number of inflammatory conditions (Kalliomaki et al., 2001), creating an environment ripe with the potential for the acquisition of adverse health conditions that have inflammatory origins. For example, deviations in intestinal microbiota may precede the development of overweight and obesity, as systemic low-grade inflammation and aberrant local gut microbiota serve as contributing factors to over nutrition (Backhed et al., 2004; Fantuzzi, 2005). High levels of *Bacteroides* in the gut microbiota in animal models were shown to predispose toward increased energy storage and obesity (Backhed et al., 2004; Ley et al., 2005). Kalliomaki, Collado, Salminen, and Isolauri (2008) demonstrated that bifidobacterial numbers were higher in infancy and *Staphylococcus aureus* was lower in infancy for 7-year-old normal-weight children compared with children developing overweight. This implies that high numbers of *Bifidobacteria* and low numbers of *Staphylococcus aureus* during infancy, as seen in breastfed infants, may confer a degree of protection against overweight and obesity. Because adiposity is characterized by low-grade inflammation, the provision of breastmilk with its modulation of inflammatory pathways contributes to the protection of infants from the development of overweight and obesity. Infant formula has a different effect on the architecture, hydrolysis, and absorption functions in the intestine compared with breastmilk.

Infants have a functionally immature and immuno-naive gut at birth. The tight junctions of the GI mucosa take many weeks to mature and close the gut to whole proteins and pathogens. Intestinal permeability decreases faster in breastfed infants than in formula-fed infants (Catassi, Bonucci, Coppa, Carlucci, & Giorgi, 1995), with human milk accelerating the maturation of the gut barrier function while formula does not (Newburg & Walker, 2007). The open junctions and immaturity of the GI tract's mucosal barrier contribute to the acquisition of necrotizing enterocolitis (NEC), diarrheal disease, and allergy. Preterm infants are at an even higher risk when breastmilk is supplemented with infant formula. Preterm infants already experience a high risk for acquiring NEC due to their lower gastric acid production, reduced ability to break down toxins, and low levels of sIgA, which increases bacterial adherence to the intestinal mucosa. Taylor, Basile, Ebeling, & Wagner (2009) studied 62 preterm infants and demonstrated that those infants receiving greater than 75% of their diet as breastmilk had significantly lower intestinal permeability compared with formula-fed infants or those who received only small amounts of breastmilk. The dose of breastmilk became even more important over time, as more than 25% of the diet needed to be breastmilk at 30 days of age to still see a significant advantage. Preterm infants cannot fully digest carbohydrates and proteins. Undigested casein, the protein in infant formula, can function as a chemo attractant for neutrophils, exacerbating the inflammatory response and opening the tight junctions between intestinal epithelial cells, disrupting the integrity of the epithelium barrier, and allowing the delivery of whole bacteria, endotoxin, and viruses directly into the bloodstream (Claud & Walker, 2001). Feeding preterm infants with infant formula may produce colonization of the intestine with pathogenic bacteria, resulting in an exaggerated inflammatory response. The sIgA from colostrum, transitional milk, and mature milk (which is absent in infant formula) coats the gut, preventing attachment and invasion of pathogens by competitively binding and neutralizing bacterial antigens. This passively provides immunity during a time of reduced neonatal gut immune function.

Free fatty acids created during the digestion of infant formula (but not breastmilk) have been shown to cause cellular death that may contribute to necrotizing enterocolitis in preterm infants. Necrotizing enterocolitis is much more likely to develop in preterm infants who are fed formula. Penn et al. (2012) "digested" infant formulas and breastmilk *in vitro* and tested for free fatty acids and whether these fatty acids killed off three types of cells involved in necrotizing enterocolitis: epithelial cells that line the intestine, endothelial cells that line blood vessels, and neutrophils that respond to inflammation. The digestion of formula led to cell death in less than five minutes in some cases, while breastmilk did not. Digestion of infant formula caused death in 47-99% of neutrophils while only 6% of them died as a result of breastmilk digestion. This overwhelming cytotoxicity of infant formula should signal clinicians that every effort should be made for breastmilk to be fed to all infants, especially preterm infants, and that formula supplementation should be avoided if possible.

Just One Bottle

It has long been known that relatively small amounts of formula supplementation of breastfed infants (one supplement per 24 hours) result in shifts from a breastfed to a formula-fed gut flora pattern (Bullen, Tearle, & Stewart, 1977). With the introduction of supplementary formula, the flora becomes almost indistinguishable from normal adult flora within 24 hours (Gerstley, Howell, & Nagel, 1932). If breastmilk were again given exclusively, it would take two to four weeks for the intestinal environment to return to a state favoring the gram-positive flora (Brown & Bosworth, 1922; Gerstley, Howell, & Nagel, 1932).

It is thought that initial sensitization to food allergens in the exclusively breastfed infant may occur from external sources, such as a single feeding of infant formula. In susceptible families breastfed infants can be sensitized to cow's milk protein by the giving of "just one bottle" (inadvertent supplementation, unnecessary supplementation, or planned supplementation) in the newborn nursery during the first three days of life (Cantani & Micera, 2005; Host 1991; Host, Husby, & Osterballe, 1988). The feeding of a cow's-milk-based infant formula as a supplement to breastfeeding in the hospital has been shown to increase the risk of cow's milk allergy, as does occasional exposure to cow's milk formula during the first eight weeks following discharge (Saarinen et al., 2000). As early as

1935, Ratner recommended that isolated exposure to cow's milk be avoided in infants fed breastmilk (Ratner, 1935). Small doses of allergens can serve to sensitize an infant to subsequent challenges compared with large doses, which induce tolerance.

Perturbations to the normal healthy colonization patterns of the gut can result in lifelong disease (Di Mauro et al., 2013). Such perturbations can be specifically caused by the use of infant formula which changes the bacterial population. Breastmilk's protective action relies mainly on its ability to modulate intestinal microflora composition during the early days of life (Guaraldi & Salvatori, 2012). The early bacterial colonizers of the infant's gut regulate the gene expression of the cells that line the digestive tract, creating a favorable environment for themselves which inhibits the growth of potentially pathogenic bacteria. Even small amounts of formula supplementation of breastfed infants will result in shifts from a breastfed microbiota pattern to a formula-fed pattern (Mackie, Sghir, & Gaskins, 1999). The prudent clinician may wish to avoid giving breastfed babies infant formula in the hospital and before gut closure occurs.

Chapter 3. Reasons for Supplementation

A host of reasons have been put forth for supplementing breastfed infants, both in-hospital and following discharge. While some indications are medically necessary, many other reasons are non-evidence-based, reflect incorrect knowledge or assumptions of both mothers and clinicians, are rooted in a laissez-faire attitude toward breastfeeding, are engaged in without consideration of potential hazards, occur due to comfort with the idea of formula feeding, and may be perceived as a normal course of infant feeding. Some of these reasons include:

Weight Loss

Concern about the potential for excessive weight loss in an exclusively breastfed infant is reasonable, but has also been used to defend the non-evidence-based prophylactic and "therapeutic" feeding of water, glucose water, and formula. It represents a significant threat to exclusive breastfeeding in the hospital and during the early days post discharge. The American Academy of Pediatrics states that an acceptable weight loss for breastfed infants during the first three to five days of life is up to 7% of the birth weight, with an evaluation for breastfeeding problems if weight loss exceeds 7% (American Academy of Pediatrics, 2012). Given the normal over-hydration status of the fetus and newborn, the typical meconium loss, and the small amounts of colostrum intake during the early days post birth, weight loss is considered a physiologically appropriate event. Knowledge deficits regarding the amount of available colostrum and the volume of milk required by newborns has led both parents and healthcare providers to supplement breastfed infants with sterile water, five percent dextrose water, 10% dextrose water, or formula in an attempt to compensate for "insufficient milk," to feed the infant "until the milk comes in," or because the infant is "too big" or "too small." Research shows that normative weight loss in breastfed infants averages about 5-7% of their birth weight in the first few days of life, generally peaking on day three after birth and recovering by day eight (Crossland, Richmond, Hudson, Smith, & Abu-Harb, 2008; Macdonald, Ross, Grant, & Young, 2003; Rodriguez et al., 2000). Clinicians become watchful and may intervene when this weight loss reaches 7-10%. Weight loss exceeding 10% of birth weight must be evaluated and addressed. Newborn weight loss in the first 24 hours was reported as a strong predictor of eventual maximum weight loss during the hospital stay (Flaherman, Kuzniewicz, et al., 2013). A weight loss greater than 4% by 24 hours was associated with a twofold increase in the odds of eventual in-hospital weight loss equal to or greater than 10% (Flaherman, Bokser, & Newman, 2010). This study did not take into account that some of the early weight loss can be accounted for by the amount of intravenous (IV) fluid received by the mother during labor, the diuresis that normally occurs during the early days post birth, and the loss of meconium. This type of weight loss can occur in the absence of any breastfeeding difficulties or deficits. Increased weight loss in breastfed infants has been associated with cesarean delivery (Manganaro, Mami, Marrone, Marseglia, & Gemelli, 2001). Among the exclusively breastfed neonates in this study, 77% of those with a weight loss of greater than 10% had been delivered by cesarean birth. Preer, Newby, and Philipp (2012) found that exclusively breastfed infants delivered by cesarean birth in the absence of labor experienced higher than expected weight loss. Infants whose mothers did not experience labor prior to the cesarean birth lost 1.2% more of their birth weight compared with infants whose mothers underwent labor before the cesarean delivery. They speculate that one reason for this could be the possibility that retained lung fluid contributed to a greater percentage of weight loss as the fluid is diuresed during the early hours and days following birth. Slower than normal clearance of lung fluid can result from the absence of labor, which slows the rapid re-absorption of fetal lung fluid seen after a vaginal birth. Clinicians will need to exercise greater vigilance in cesarean-born infants to assure extra breastfeeding support and rapid resolution of any breastfeeding problems. However, Preer and colleagues mention that if weight loss in these infants is slightly higher than expected, but the infant is latching well, transferring colostrum, and voiding and stooling adequately, then clinical concern may be reduced in this situation.

Large amounts of IV fluids are often received by laboring mothers. Fluids received by mothers during labor are rapidly equilibrated with the fetus (Carvalho & Mathias, 1994). Significant weight loss in the newborn's first days following birth may be related to a fluid shift from the mother to the fetus in the absence of breastfeeding inadequacies or pathology. Since weight loss is often the driver of interventions, such as delayed discharge or formula supplementation, it is important that clinicians take into account newborn fluid overload as a contributor to newborn weight loss. Numerous authors have demonstrated a relationship between intrapartum fluid intake and neonatal weight loss:

- Mulder, Johnson, and Baker (2010) studied 53 breastfeeding infants who lost either less than or greater than 7% of their birth weight during the hospital stay. Infants losing greater than 7%

of their birth weight were shown to have significantly more total voids and a higher breastfeeding frequency than infants losing less than 7% of their birth weight. A logistic regression analysis showed that total voids was the only significant predictor of a 7% or greater weight loss. In the absence of other indicators of ineffective breastfeeding, infants losing greater than 7% of their birth weight may be experiencing a physiologic diuresis not related to their breastfeeding behaviors.

- Lamp and Macke (2010) also showed that a strong predictor of neonatal weight loss within the first 48 hours was the average number of wet diapers.

- Okumus et al. (2011) reported that postnatal weight loss was higher in infants whose mothers had a cesarean delivery and epidural analgesia compared with infants whose mothers experienced a vaginal delivery. Postnatal weight losses were correlated with the amount of IV fluid volume infused into the mother during the last six hours prior to delivery.

- Chantry, Nommsen-Rivers, Peerson, Cohen, and Dewey (2011) reported that the relative risk of infants losing greater than 10% of their birth weight tripled when women had a positive fluid balance of greater than 200 ml/hour during the intrapartum period. Number of voids during the first four hours following birth were greater for infants whose mothers had a positive fluid balance that exceeded 200 ml/hour.

- Watson, Hodnett, Armson, Davies, and Watt-Watson (2012) showed that weight loss in infants whose mothers received greater than 2500 ml of IV fluid during labor was significantly higher than in infants whose mothers received lower IV fluid volumes. The authors recommend that clinicians take into account the volumes of IV fluid infused during the intrapartum period when assessing contributions to early newborn weight loss in the first 48 hours of life.

- Noel-Weiss, Woodend, Peterson, Gibb, and Groll (2011) demonstrated a correlation between neonatal urine output, the amount of infused maternal IV fluids, and newborn weight loss. For mothers who had 1200 ml or less IV fluids, the average percentage of newborn weight loss at 60 hours was 5.51%. The group receiving more than 1200 ml total fluids had infants who averaged a 6.93% weight loss. Late onset of lactogenesis II showed a positive correlation to the percentage of newborn weight loss. These authors discuss that newborns may have an artificially high reference point for newborn weight loss when using birth weight as the reference. Resetting the baseline weight to a point after diuresis has occurred and the weight has stabilized may provide a more accurate way to determine actual weight loss. A frequency analysis of percentage weight loss was conducted to contrast two possible outcomes using a baseline of the actual birth weight compared to weight 24 hours later, after diuresis had occurred in the infants in this study. Using a 24-hour baseline weight, 2.3% of infants lost between 7-10% of their birth weight, with none losing more than 10%. However, when using the actual weight at birth as a baseline, 33% of newborns lost between 7-10% of their birth weight and 7.3% lost more than 10%. The authors suggest that weight at 24 hours is a better reference point at which to start monitoring newborn weight loss, rather than actual weight at birth.

• Hirth, Weitkamp, and Dwivedi (2012) demonstrated that maternal average IV milliliter of fluid per hour given during labor positively correlated with maximum infant weight loss. For every 1% increase in average ml per hour of IV fluid during labor, the infant maximum weight loss percent will increase by 0.0077. The authors provided a sample calculation as an example which showed the following:

> "…assume a 5 percent infant maximum weight loss, and a change in average IV mL per hour from 150 to 225 (a 50 percent increase). Then maximum weight-loss percent would be predicted to increase by 0.0077 x 50, which is 0.39, giving a total maximum weight-loss percent of 5.39 (5 + 0.39)."

Breastfeeding is not necessarily a risk factor for greater neonatal weight loss if weight loss is monitored, breastfeeding is repeatedly assessed and appropriately supported, and careful supplementation (preferably with expressed colostrum) is judiciously used to treat excess weight loss (Davanzo, Cannioto, Ronfani, Monasta, & Demarini, 2013).

Water or formula supplementation of breastfed infants in the hospital does not necessarily prevent weight loss (Herrera, 1984; Shrago, 1987). Bertini, Dani, Tronchin, and Rubaltelli (2001) reported on the relationship between weight loss and supplementation of breastfed infants with formula. In this study those breastfed infants supplemented with formula lost significantly more weight than exclusively breastfed infants or exclusively bottle-fed infants. In a chart audit of 74 mothers, Glover (1990) showed that breastfed infants who received glucose water demonstrated a larger percentage of birth weight loss (2.43-15.87%) compared with unsupplemented breastfed newborns (2.97-7.48%). Weight loss in infants supplemented with sterile water or five percent glucose water is consistent with the lower caloric density of these fluids compared with colostrum, transitional, and mature milk. One ounce of five percent dextrose water contains five calories, one ounce of 10% dextrose water contains ten calories, and one ounce of colostrum contains 18–20 calories. For each ounce of five percent dextrose water consumed by a breastfed infant, his or her caloric intake is reduced by approximately two thirds. The risk of excess infant weight loss has been shown to be 7.1 times greater if the mother has delayed onset of milk production (Dewey et al., 2003). Neifert (1998, 1999) recommended that weight loss of 8% or more from birth weight, failure to surpass birth weight by two weeks of age, or failure to commence weight gain of approximately 28 g per day by five days of age warrant further investigation.

Healthy full-term newborns have an abundance of extracellular and extravascular water. Total body water declines abruptly after birth as the infant transitions from an aquatic environment to a terrestrial or dry environment. Fluid moves from the intracellular compartment to the extracelluar fluid compartment leading to a water loss of about one to three percent of their birth weight on a daily basis for the first couple of days. Caution, therefore, is necessary in the use of water supplementation of newborns to avoid fluid overload. Water intoxication with seizures was reported in a breastfed infant who was given 675 ml (22.5 oz) of supplementary glucose water during the 24 hours before transfer from the maternity unit to the neonatal intensive care unit (Ruth-Sanchez & Greene, 1997). Neonates born to mothers who have received dextrose-containing IV fluids during labor can experience enough of a fluid shift to skew weight loss calculations toward the appearance of a clinical problem of excessive loss of birth weight, when what is really taking place is a diuresis of excess fluid (Keppler, 1988). Dahlenburg, Burnell, and Braybrook (1980) examined the serum sodium levels in newborns whose mothers received IV fluids containing five percent dextrose and oxytocin. The mean sodium levels were significantly lower in the infants whose mothers had IV fluids compared with those who did not. Percentage of weight loss in infants whose mothers received IV fluids was 6.17% ± 3.36% compared with 4.07% ± 2.20% weight loss in infants whose mothers did not receive IV fluids during labor. While dextrose solutions are rarely used on current labor and delivery units, both maternal and neonatal serum sodium concentrations can be significantly decreased when dextrose is used only as the diluent (rather than normal saline) for oxytocin infusion in induction or augmentation of labor (Higgins, Gleeson, Holohan, Cooney, & Darling, 1996; Stratton, Stronge, & Boylan, 1995). Most hospitals have abandoned the use of sugar water for newborn infants, as it is no longer an evidence-based practice. However, results of the 2007 mPINC survey conducted by the Centers for Disease Control and Prevention revealed that 30% of surveyed hospitals reported giving feedings of glucose water to newborns.[12]

Breastfed infants whose mothers received epidurals have been shown to lose more weight in the first 24 hours than infants whose mothers did not have an epidural. Merry and Montgomery (2000) reported that the average weight loss in the first day for infants whose mothers had an epidural was 226 g (8 oz) compared with 142 g (5 oz) in a non-epidural group. It is possible that administration of IV fluids during labor, which is more common in women receiving analgesia or anesthesia, could initially increase the hydration status of the newborn, with a subsequent rapid weight loss mimicking underfeeding. Once started, water supplementation can often remain prevalent in the first month of life, even in exclusively breastfed infants (Scariati, Grummer-Strawn, & Fein, 1997). A side effect of large volumes of intrapartum IV fluids is the associated decrease in oncotic pressure, which may subsequently increase breast and areolar engorgement, interfering with infant latching and milk transfer, a prelude to weight loss (Cotterman, 2004).

Martens and Romphf (2007) demonstrated that several factors significantly increased the percentage of weight loss in newborn infants. These included birth weight, female gender, epidural use, and a longer hospital stay. In this study supplemented breastfed infants lost more weight than exclusively breastfed newborns, as did those whose mothers had epidurals during labor and delivery. Formula-fed infants lost approximately 3% of birth weight, substantially less than a breastfed infant who actually represents the norm. The authors speculated that formula-fed infants (who were 111 g heavier than breastfed infants during the first three days postpartum) may be at risk for overfeeding in the early days. These infants were in reality being over-fed at a time when early feeding experiences could be critical to metabolic imprinting and the development of future overweight or obesity (Lucas, 1998; de Moura, Lisboa, & Passos, 2008). Unnecessary or unphysiological amounts of formula supplements may predispose infants to later overweight problems. Stettler et al. (2005) found a 28% increased

---

12   http://www.cdc.gov/mmwr/preview/mmwrhtml/mm5723a1.htm?s_cid=mm5723a1_e

risk of obesity in adults for every 100 g of weight an infant gained in his or her first week of life.

In a study of 205 late preterm infants, three factors were found to be highly associated with the risk of developing significant newborn weight loss: having a mother with previous negative breastfeeding experience, exposure to phototherapy, and cesarean delivery (Kusuma, Agrawal, Kumar, Narang, & Prasad, 2009).

Caglar, Ozer, and Altugan (2006) reported that infants with a weight loss of more than 10% were more likely to be from primiparous mothers, to experience a delay in receiving their first breastfeeding, to pass less than four stools per day, and to have uric acid crystals in their diaper. This alerts the clinician to the need by first-time mothers for extra vigilance, ensuring that the infant is swallowing milk and that the mother knows how to tell when the infant is swallowing.

Clinical Implications

Weight change patterns help clinicians identify situations of concern, but interventions such as supplementing breastfed infants with formula should not be based solely on maintaining an infant's weight within pre-established norms (Noel-Weiss, Courant, & Woodend, 2008). Often, the underlying assumption is that weight loss is due to insufficient milk supply or ineffective milk transfer, but other confounding factors may also be present. Birthing practices, hospital routines, maternal IV fluid volume, birth experiences, cesarean delivery, and late preterm birth, are also associated with weight loss. These should not be overlooked during weight loss assessments. Seldom is the amount of stooling and voiding entered into the equation of neonatal weight loss. Prevention of excessive weight loss begins with optimal breastfeeding management, observations of early feeding to assure infant swallowing of colostrum, monitoring urine and especially stooling output, weighing of the infant prior to discharge and by two to three days of age, and increased vigilance in infants and mothers with known risk factors for excessive newborn weight loss.

Dehydration

Dehydration and hypernatremia, while not common in breastfed infants, still occasionally occur as isolated incidents. Most reports are of case studies or a case series with the common factor of exclusive breastfeeding seen in the majority of the subjects. Prophylactic or routine administration of water or formula to breastfed infants to prevent dehydration has not been shown to be necessary. Dehydration is unlikely to occur in full-term healthy newborns who are able to successfully transfer colostrum and milk from the breast and who are given ample opportunities to do so when they demonstrate feeding readiness cues. Rodriguez et al. (2000) calculated the loss of total body water and body solids during the first three days of life. The percentage of total body water actually increased, indicating adequate hydration, whereas the weight of the infant decreased due to the greater loss of body solids (stool), not the loss of total body water. Infants who pass several large meconium stools during the first 24-48 hours may give the appearance of not being adequately fed or hydrated, but do not require intervention unless other feeding parameters are unacceptable.

Renal function is unique in the newborn and differs from that in older children and adults. The normal neonate has 6-44 ml of urine in the bladder at birth. Approximately 17% of newborns void directly after delivery, 92% by 24 hours, and 99% by 48 hours. Newborns tend to be oliguretic (low urinary output) for the first day because of high circulating levels of maternal anti-diuretic hormone after birth. If the infant has voided at delivery, then urine output in the first 24 hours can be misleading (Black, 2001) because another void may not become apparent until many hours later. The full-term infant typically creates a urine volume of 15-60 ml per 24 hours. Voiding size is 19.3 ml, with urine formation ranging from 0.5 to 5.0 mg/kg per hour at all gestational ages. Normal neonates void two to six times per day during the first 48 hours of life and 5-25 times daily thereafter. Voiding during the first two to three days reflects the depletion of the infant's extravascular and extracellular reserve and may be reflected in diaper counts of one to two diapers, with amounts increasing as lactogenesis II occurs on days three to four. Urine output increases rapidly after this time.

Hypernatremic dehydration, however, can represent the extreme spectrum of a deteriorating clinical situation (Neifert, 2001). An infant who is unable to transfer milk and a mother who has a depleted milk supply, delayed lactogenesis II, underproduction, or any number of other risk factors (Tables 3.1 and 3.2) should be evaluated promptly to avoid true infant dehydration.

Fever and hypernatremia are often found in neonates with excessive weight loss. In low-risk, full-term infants, fever with no other symptoms during the first days is frequently related to dehydration and problems with breastfeeding. Jaundice and poor sucking may be the major presenting symptoms (Unal, Arhan, Kara, Uncu, & Alliefendioglu, 2008).

TABLE 3.1. Maternal Risk Factors for Infant Dehydration

- Previous insufficient milk or underweight, breastfed infant
- Flat or inverted nipples affecting infant latch or milk removal
- Breast anomalies such as markedly asymmetrical, tubular, or hypoplastic breasts
- Excessive, prolonged, or unrelieved breast engorgement
- Previous breast surgery (periareolar incisions, abscess)
- Cracked, bleeding nipples or persistent nipple pain
- Perinatal complications (hemorrhage, hypertension, infection)
- Pre-existing maternal conditions (overweight, obesity, diabetes, endocrine disorders such as Polycystic Ovary Syndrome)
- Lack of previous breastfeeding experience or primiparous
- Maternal age older than 37 years
- Labor and delivery variations (vacuum extraction, labor medications, prolonged labor)
- Cesarean delivery

Hypernatremia can cause disruption in the blood-brain barrier, facilitating the diffusion of bilirubin into the brain. This can lead to a worsening cycle of dehydration, jaundice, and hypernatremia. Often, jaundice is the presenting complaint along with a weight loss of greater than 7% (Uras, Karadag, Dogan, Tonbul, & Tatli, 2007). Hypernatremic dehydration may be difficult to recognize clinically, but weight loss and inadequate stooling are sensitive indicators of dehydration (Moritz, Manole, Bogen, & Ayus, 2005). Weight loss is strongly associated with hypernatremia. Breastfeeding difficulty and weight loss are commonly present in infants with hypernatremia or dehydration (Oddie, Craven, Deakin, Westman, & Scally, 2013). Scant bowel output during the first five days after delivery or delayed transition of bowel movements to a yellow color are markers for immediate follow-up (Shrago, Reifsnider, & Insel, 2006). Konetzny, Bucher, and Arlettaz (2009) found that infants born by cesarean section had a 3.4 times higher risk for hypernatremia than those born vaginally, reminding clinicians that these babies may need closer follow-up both during the hospital stay and post discharge. Weighing infants at 72-96 hours after birth helps in the early recognition of hypernatremic dehydration and reduces the potential extent of the dehydration and hypernatremia while preserving breastfeeding (Iyer et al., 2008). Mothers should be provided with information such as that seen in Figure 3.1 that addresses feeding adequacy and alerts them to when they should consult a healthcare provider (Livingstone, Willis, Abdel-Wareth, Thiessen, & Lockitch, 2000).

TABLE 3.2. Early Infant Breastfeeding Risk Factors for Dehydration

- Gestational age (preterm and late preterm)
- Small for gestation age, intrauterine growth retardation, low birth weight
- Separation from mother for more than 24 hours
- Oral anatomical defects (cleft lip/palate, micrognathia, macroglossia, ankyloglossia, bubble palate)
- Neurological or neuromotor problems (Down syndrome, dysfunctional sucking)
- Sucking variations (non-sustained, non-nutritive, disorganized, weak)
- Hyperbilirubinemia, especially if using phototherapy
- Multiple births
- Systemic illness (increased oxygen requirement, cardiac defect, infection)
- Difficulty latching correctly to one or both breasts
- Sleepy infant with poor or subtle feeding cues
- Irritability, fretfulness, apparent hunger after feeds
- Excessive pacifier use
- Weight loss of more than 7% of birth weight
- Not passing yellow, breastmilk stools by four days of age; fewer than four sizable stools per day between four days and four weeks of age
- Fewer than six clear voids per day by four days of age
- Appearance of urate crystals in the diaper after three days of age
- Failure to exceed birth weight by 10-14 days of age
- Failure to begin weight gain of approximately 28 g/day after day four or five

Sources: Adapted from Neifert, M.R. (2001). Prevention of breastfeeding tragedies. *Pediatric Clinics of North America, 48*,273–297; Walker, M. (1989). Functional assessment of infant breastfeeding patterns. *Birth, 16,* 140–147.

Dehydration and hypernatremia are much less likely to occur when infants are born in hospitals with the Baby Friendly designation (Oddie et al., 2013). Hospitals with policies that specifically support exclusive breastfeeding and engage in such practices can help protect against the development of severe feeding difficulties or omissions in care that can lead to aberrant breastfeeding outcomes, such as dehydration and hypernatremia (Mikiel-Kostra & Mazur, 1999). Infant weight loss during the hospital stay can be exacerbated by outdated and non-evidence-based maternity unit care practices. Clinical practices at a Baby Friendly designated hospital that support and optimize breastfeeding have been shown to be associated with

Breastfeeding Checklist for Newborns

Post on your refrigerator or on the back of your bathroom door.

Baby's birth date and time: _____

Your baby will be 4 days old on _____

Baby's birth weight: _____

Baby's discharge weight: _____
(It's normal to lose up to 7% from birth.)

Baby's weight at check-up 2 days after discharge: _____

Baby's second week weight: _____
(Baby should have regained his birth weight by 14 days.)

Important Numbers:

Pediatrician: _____

OB-GYN Doctor: _____

Lactation Consultant: _____

Find more support near you at Zipmilk.org –
just enter your zip code.

Some signs that breastfeeding is going well:

☐ Your baby is breastfeeding at least 8 times every 24 hours.

☐ Your baby has at least 4 yellow bowel movements every 24 hours by day 4.

☐ You can hear your baby gulping or swallowing at feedings.

☐ Once your baby latches on, your nipples do not hurt when your baby nurses.

☐ Your baby is receiving only breast milk.

Check in with your pediatrician's office or lactation consultant if:

☐ Your baby is having fewer than 4 poopy diapers per 24 hours by day 4.

☐ There are any red stains in the diaper after day 3. (It can be normal in the first 3 days.)

☐ Your baby is still having black tarry bowel movements on day 4.

☐ Your baby is not breastfeeding at least 8 times every 24 hours.

☐ You can't hear your baby gulping or swallowing, or you can't tell.

☐ Your nipples hurt during feeding, even after the baby is first latched on.

☐ Your baby does not seem satisfied after most feedings.

It is your responsibility to contact your baby's doctor
to schedule visits, including a visit 2 days after going home.

**Do not wait to call your baby's doctor or the
lactation consultant if you think breastfeeding
is not going well.**

© MBC 2006. Credit to Nebose-Wakefield Hospital Lactation Department

*Massachusetts
Breastfeeding
Coalition*

www.massbfc.org | zipmilk.org

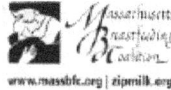

Figure 3.1. Breastfeeding Checklist for Newborns

Source: Courtesy of the Massachusetts Breastfeeding Coalition, www.massbfc.org.

a moderate and physiologically normal weight loss in exclusively and mainly breastfed infants (Grossman, Chaudhuri, Feldman-Winter, & Merewood, 2012).

In the past there was some thought that high sodium levels in the breastmilk of mothers whose infants were hypernatremic contributed to the acquisition of the condition. If breastfeeding mothers have infants who are unable to establish effective feeding, then as milk production decreases sodium content of the milk increases. Thus, the normal physiological decrease in breastmilk sodium concentration does not occur (Morton, 1994) and the sodium concentration remains high, mimicking the weaning process. High sodium levels in breastmilk are not the cause of hypernatremic dehydration, they are the result of the cause.

Clinical implications

Prevention of dehydration and hypernatremia can be accomplished with knowledge of the major contributors to these conditions, assurance of successful milk transfer, and close monitoring post discharge of mothers and infants at high risk for these conditions. Special vigilance is in order for conditions that create a prolonged colostral phase, i.e., delayed lactogenesis II, maternal obesity, maternal diabetes, cesarean delivery, primiparous mother, infant latch and sucking difficulties, and late preterm infant. Care plans for these situations may include more frequent breastfeedings, use of alternate massage to improve milk transfer, hand expression of colostrum and pumping, and supplementation with expressed colostrum and breastmilk.

Hyperbilirubinemia (Jaundice)

Prevention of hyperbilirubinemia (jaundice) is often cited as a reason for recommending formula supplementation, as is the misconception that bilirubin can be flushed out of the system by increasing water intake. The imbalance between the production and elimination of bilirubin results in varying levels of hyperbilirubinemia in most newborns. At birth normal, healthy, full-term infants have a cord total serum bilirubin concentration of about 1.5 mg/dl (25.5 μmol/L). This increases in the early days to a mean peak of approximately 5.5 mg/dl (93.5 μmol/L) by the third day in African America and Caucasian infants and 10 mg/dl (170 μmol/L) in infants of Asian origin (Halamek & Stevenson, 1996). Breastfed infants of Asian origin (Japanese, Korean, and Chinese), as well as breastfed Navajo Indian and Alaska Native newborns, appear to have exaggerated physiological jaundice independent of feeding method (Johnson, 1992). While some degree of hyperbilirubinemia is a normal physiological phenomenon, its severity can be influenced by genetic factors. A particular gene mutation associated with hyperbilirubinemia is very common among Asian infants, especially breastfed ones (Akaba et al., 1998; Chou et al., 2011). Asian infants carrying a particular genetic mutation (G71R mutation of UGT1A1) and experiencing inadequate breastfeeding with a greater than 5% weight loss may present with a significant increase in serum bilirubin levels (Sato et al., 2013; Ishihara et al., 2001). Effective breastfeeding could help compensate for the genetic predisposing factor (G71R mutation of UGT1A1) to hyperbilirubinemia in Asian breastfed infants.

Breastfed and formula-fed infants have been shown to have differing bilirubin patterns, with breastfed infants experiencing a more gradual decline in bilirubin levels or with bilirubin concentration reaching a second peak around the 10th day of life (Itoh, Kondo, Kusaka, Isobe, & Onishi, 2001; Gartner & Herschel, 2001). A number of factors can contribute to elevated bilirubin levels in newborn infants:

- Feeding frequency and bilirubin levels are inversely associated in the first three days of life. Infants fed eight times or less per 24 hours had significantly higher bilirubin levels on day three (9.3 mg/dl) than did infants fed more than eight times per 24 hours (6.5 mg/dl) (De Carvalho, Klaus, & Merkatz, 1982). As the frequency of breastfeeding decreases, the incidence and levels of bilirubin increase over the first week of life. Yamauchi and Yamanouchi (1990) looked at the frequency of breastfeeding during the first 24 hours and the incidence of bilirubin levels exceeding 15 mg/dl at six days. Infants who fed 9-11 times per day had a 0% rate, those feeding seven to eight times per 24 hours had a rate of 11.8%, those feeding five to six times per 24 hours yielded a 15.2% rate, three to four times showed a 24.5% rate, and infants fed less frequently than that showed a 28.1% rate of significant jaundice. Okechukwu and Okolo (2006) showed an inverse relationship between the frequency of feedings and serum bilirubin levels on days three and seven of life. The more breastfeedings received by the infant, the lower the bilirubin levels. Also seen was a positive correlation between frequent feedings and the early passage of meconium during the first 24 hours.

- Water supplementation has an inverse relationship with bilirubin levels and has been shown long ago to contribute to higher bilirubin levels rather than prevent or ameliorate them. The more water given to breastfed infants, the higher their bilirubin levels (Nicoll, Ginsburg, & Tripp, 1982). Supplementary water does not prophylactically prevent or lower bilirubin levels (De Carvalho, Hall, & Harvey, 1981).

- Meconium passage is also related to bilirubin levels, as meconium is laden with bilirubin. As stooling volume increases, serum bilirubin levels decrease. Early initiation and more frequent breastfeeding avoid delayed fecal bilirubin clearance (De Carvalho, Robertson, & Klaus, 1985).

- High bilirubin levels are related to significant weight loss in the newborn. The risk of developing severe hyperbilirubinemia has been reported to be four times greater for infants with significant weight loss compared with infants who experience normal physiological weight loss (Salas et al., 2009). Lack of calories from inefficient breastfeeding contributes to delayed gastrointestinal motility, increasing the entero-hepatic circulation of bilirubin. One study showed that an 8% or greater weight loss after 48 hours and an 11% or greater weight loss after 72 hours significantly increased the risk for hyperbilirubinemia (Chang et al., 2012). Birth weight loss percentage cutoff values that were clinically useful in predicting significant hyperbilirubinemia at 72 hours were reported to be 4.48% on day one, 7.60% by day two, and 8.15% by day three (Yang et al., 2013). These numbers did not take into account weight loss from diuresis of excess fluid, nor weight loss from meconium stooling. While these weight loss percentage numbers are not an ideal predictor of significant hyperbilirubinemia, they may be useful as an indicator that more intense breastfeeding interventions could be necessary.

- Bertini et al. (2001) reported a significant correlation between breastfed infants with elevated bilirubin levels (bilirubin levels > 12.9 mg/dl; 221 mmol/L) and supplementary feeding. Breastfed infants did not have excessive bilirubin levels in the first days of life, except for a subpopulation that showed a greater weight loss than the mean. Jaundice was not associated with breastfeeding per se, but rather with an increased weight loss after birth subsequent to fasting, suggesting the important role of caloric intake in the regulation of serum bilirubin. Thus, breastfed infants who receive low-calorie supplements in place of colostrum and breastfed infants who are unable to transfer colostrum and subsequently receive supplementation show much higher levels of bilirubin. Among the other conditions favoring jaundice (ABO blood incompatibility, supplementary feeding, weight loss, and Asian ethnicity) was the finding that infants born by vacuum extraction were at a high risk for exaggerated jaundice. Seventeen percent of vacuum-extracted infants had total serum bilirubin values exceeding 12.9 mg/dl. This finding is consistent with the development of scalp or brain bleeding associated with vacuum extraction (Rubaltelli, 1968; Werner et al., 2011).

- Oxytocin exposure during labor and delivery has been identified as a risk factor for hyperbilirubinemia (Keren et al., 2005). This exposure may have some direct effect on neonatal bilirubin metabolism.

Clinical Implications

Once formed, bilirubin cannot be diluted or flushed out by giving additional water. Bilirubin is conjugated by the liver, and almost all of it is excreted via the bile into the stools. Water is not a limiting or facilitating factor in bilirubin metabolism. Giving additional water decreases breastmilk and caloric intake, reduces breast stimulation, increases the risk for insufficient milk, increases bilirubin levels, and is counterproductive to establishing breastfeeding and adequate lactation. Water supplements may result in adequate hydration, but create simultaneous caloric deprivation, contributing to the very situation the supplements were supposed to avoid. The American Academy of Pediatrics (2012) recommends against routine supplementation of non-dehydrated breastfed infants with water or dextrose water. In spite of the data and recommendations to the contrary, the mPINC survey found that 30% of facilities gave feedings of glucose water and 15% gave water to breastfed infants, practices known to be detrimental to breastfeeding (Centers for Disease Control and Prevention, 2008). Dextrose/water or formula supplements may substitute for clinical interventions necessary to prevent excessive bilirubin levels from developing pre and post discharge. Rather than water or formula supplements as a first-line approach, clinicians can take a preventive approach to hyperbilirubinemia (Bhutani & Johnson, 2009) that includes optimal breastfeeding support (making sure that mothers know when their infant is swallowing milk), referral to an International Board Certified Lactation Consultant (IBCLC) in-hospital for breastfeeding problems and following discharge, facilitation of risk assessment for hyperbilirubinemia in the hospital through use of a bilirubin nomogram, more intense monitoring of infants at increased risk (such as late preterm infants), and a follow-up appointment with the infant's physician within 48 hours of discharge. If a supplement is necessary, the first choice would be mother's own milk or pasteurized donor milk. If formula must be used, then a hydrolyzed formula rather than a standard cow's-milk-based formula would be a better choice. A hydrolyzed formula facilitates beta-glucuronidase inhibition and results in increased fecal bilirubin excretion (Gourley, Li, Kreamer, & Kosorok, 2005). Beta-glucuronidase is an enzyme found in breastmilk that converts conjugated bilirubin to unconjugated bilirubin for reabsorption rather than facilitating excretion, contributing to jaundice.

Hypoglycemia

Hypoglycemia is a common metabolic concern in the newborn infant and represents a continuum of blood glucose concentration, falling immediately after delivery and rising thereafter. Hypoglycemia is not a single number.

Transient hypoglycemia in the first three hours after birth is normal with spontaneous recovery. Hypoglycemia (or the potential risk for hypoglycemia) represents a frequent reason for supplementing the breastfed newborn. A major physiological challenge for newborns is to establish and regulate their own metabolic processes following birth, including the self-regulation of glucose metabolism when this function is no longer performed by the maternal placental unit. A quarter of a century ago, newborns were routinely fed nothing by mouth for 6-12 hours after birth or longer, with many newborns receiving nothing by mouth for the first 24 hours. This practice reflected a number of non-evidence-based assumptions about the early nutritional requirements of newborns. Inappropriate supplementation trends persist today due to a lack of consensus on what constitutes hypoglycemia, misunderstanding of neonatal glucose metabolism, and uncertainty about when to intervene. After delivery the maternal glucose supply to the infant is abruptly withdrawn, causing a self-limiting decline in the infant's blood sugar for about the first three hours of life (Srinivasan, Pildes, Cattamanchi, Voora, & Lilien, 1986). Blood glucose concentrations as low as 30 mg/dl are commonly seen in healthy newborns during the first one to two hours following birth. Such low blood glucose concentrations are usually transient and asymptomatic. The infant must then initiate counter-regulatory compensation through three processes, plus begin the formation of alternative brain fuels (Williams, 1997):

1. Glycolysis, the conversion of glucose to lactate and pyruvate

2. Glycogenolysis, the release of glycogen from body stores to form glucose

3. Gluconeogenesis, the production of glucose by the liver and kidneys from substrates such as fatty acids and amino acids

During this initial period of low blood glucose following delivery, the infant generates additional sources of fuel for the brain, including ketone bodies derived from a brisk ketogenic response to low blood glucose levels through fatty acid mobilization. As an adaptive response, breastfed infants experiencing the initial low blood glucose concentrations following delivery will generate high concentrations of ketone bodies, a response that is blunted by supplementation with formula (De Rooy & Hawdon, 2002). Early feeding of human milk/colostrum serves an important purpose relative to glucose homeostasis. It enhances the process of gluconeogenesis by providing amino acid precursors, by making available the fatty acids that facilitate the formation of an enzyme critical to ketogenesis, and by furnishing lactose that minimizes insulin secretion. Feeding either five percent or 10 percent glucose water in the immediate period after birth increases insulin secretion (which suppresses gluconeogenesis), decreases secretion of glucagon (a hormone that stimulates the liver to change stored glycogen to glucose and encourages the use of fats and amino acids for energy production), and delays the natural gluconeogenesis and ketogenic processes (Eidelman, 2001). In an elegant interplay of metabolic adaptation, the breastfed term infants who lose the most weight have the highest ketone body concentrations (Hawdon, Ward-Platt, & Aynsley-Green, 1992; Swenne, Ewald, Gustafsson, Sandberg, & Ostenson, 1994). This suggests that ketogenesis is an adaptive response to a temporarily low nutrient intake during the time it takes for the infant to successfully establish feeding at the breast (Cornblath et al., 2000).

Formula and breastfed infants demonstrate different patterns of serum glucose concentrations. Hawdon, Ward-Platt, and Aynsley-Green (1992) reported a mean of 3.6 mmol/L (58 mg/dl), with a range of 1.5-5.3 mmol/L (27-95 mg/dl), in breastfed infants and a mean of 4.0 mmol/L (72 mg/dl), with a range of 2.5-6.2 mmol/L (45-111 mg/dl), in formula-fed infants. None of the breastfed infants became symptomatic, and all showed significant increases in ketone bodies. Only the interval between feedings was correlated with glucose concentrations, reinforcing the recommendation for frequent breastfeeding. Considerable controversy exists regarding the actual definition of hypoglycemia (Rozance, 2013), with some current definitions not being applicable to breastfed infants because these infants can tolerate lower plasma glucose levels (Cornblath, Schwartz, Aynsley-Green, & Lloyd, 1990). Statistical rather than functional blood glucose levels have been described for hypoglycemia cut-off points that are the lower limits of normal. These distinctions are based on serum or plasma glucose concentrations, which are 10-15 percent higher than in whole blood and do not distinguish between breastfed and formula-fed infants. Some studies use very high glucose concentration cut-off points, inflating the incidence of hypogylcemia in normal, healthy, full-term infants.

Symptomatic hypoglycemia is the association of clinical signs (which can be vague and nonspecific) and blood glucose concentrations of less than arbitrary level. Healthy, normal, full-term infants do not develop symptomatic hypoglycemia simply as a result of underfeeding (Williams, 1997) and do not require routine monitoring of blood glucose levels (Eidelman, 2001). The use of bedside screening tests using reagent strips can have as high as a 20% rate of false positives (i.e., normoglycemic infants labeled erroneously as hypoglycemic) (Holtrop, Madison, Kiechle, Karcher, & Batton, 1990; Reynolds & Davies, 1993). Laboratory determinations of blood glucose concentrations should be conducted to confirm the results of bedside measurements before supplementing a breastfed infant with formula. Hypoglycemia is minimized in breastfed infants who are fed early, often, and exclusively and who are actually and adequately transferring milk (colostrum) that is confirmed by documenting swallowing. Early breastfeeding is not precluded simply because an infant meets the criteria for glucose monitoring (Wight, Marinelli, & Academy of Breastfeeding Medicine Protocol Committee, 2006). Some maternity units supplement normal, healthy, full-term infants as if they were high risk, using specific glucose levels that may inappropriately call for supplementing infants who have no medical need. Maternity units should not use glucose measurements adapted for sick infants, such as in the S.T.A.B.L.E. program (http://www.stableprogram.org/index.php), a program for post-resuscitation/pre-transport stabilization care of sick infants. Gross overfeeding of breastfed infants with infant formula to prevent or ameliorate low blood sugar levels may unintentionally result in long-term problems. Screening should be restricted to at-risk and symptomatic infants, with symptomatic infants receiving intravenous glucose therapy, not forced feedings (Wight, 2006). The risk for and incidence of hypoglycemia may actually be increasing as maternal factors known to contribute to neonatal hypoglycemia are increasing. These include obesity, diabetes, increasing maternal age, and poor economic conditions (Harris, Weston, & Harding, 2012).

The American Academy of Pediatrics provides a practical guide for screening and management of hypoglycemia in the four groups where asymptomatic hypoglycemia is most likely to occur (Adamkin & Committee on Fetus and Newborn, 2011). It reminds clinicians that any approach to hypoglycemia management should not unnecessarily disrupt breastfeeding.

Clinical Implications

Breastfeeding protocols and caretaking activities during the hours after delivery should be designed to proactively reduce the likelihood of inducing or exacerbating hypoglycemia. Chertok, Raz, Shoham, Haddad, and Wiznitzer (2009) found that infants of mothers with gestational diabetes who were breastfed immediately following birth had a significantly lower rate of borderline hypoglycemia than those not fed in the early postpartum period. They also had significantly higher mean blood glucose levels compared with those not breastfed immediately after delivery, and also had a mean blood glucose level that was higher than those infants who were formula-fed for their first feed. An infant who misses this early opportunity to breastfeed does not require supplementation, nor does a healthy full-term breastfeeding infant require routine blood glucose monitoring (Adamkin & Committee on Fetus and Newborn, 2011).

Early breastfeeding when the infant is swallowing colostrum helps facilitate glycemic stability in infants, especially in those born to diabetic mothers. It is in the best interests of the infant to assure that effective breastfeeding takes places as soon as possible after delivery and to make certain that the infant is swallowing colostrum at this time. Prevention activities also include the following:

- Breastfeed frequently, on cue, before sustained crying occurs, and avoid long intervals between feedings. Based on the newborn stomach capacity, gastric emptying time of human milk, and neonatal sleep cycles, Bergman (2013) recommends hourly feedings at this time to avoid stressing the infant and contributing to hypoglycemia. Small, frequent feedings provide the newborn with a constant supply of lactose, avoiding the stress of sympathetic nervous system activation of glycogenolysis (Brodows, Pi-Sunyer, & Campbell, 1975).

- Infants separated from their mothers have lower body temperatures, cry more, and have decreased blood glucose levels (Christensson et al.,1992; Durand et al., 1997). Christensson et al. (1992) reported that newborn infants separated from their mothers had blood sugar levels that were 10 mg/dl lower than infants kept in skin-to-skin contact with their mothers at 90 minutes following birth. Environmental stress, such as hypothermia, can increase the energy demands of a newborn, which could exceed the infant's capacity to generate energy substrate (Kaplan & Eidelman, 1985). Separation from the mother activates neonatal stress responses that further expend calories faster than they can be replaced (Winberg, 2005). Walters, Boggs, Ludington-Hoe, Price, and Morrison (2007) demonstrated that healthy term infants placed skin-to-skin within one minute of birth had temperatures that rose and blood glucose levels in a satisfactory range (43-85 mg/dl), even in infants who had not fed before the study's glucose measurement at 60 minutes after birth (43-118 mg/dl).

  - Keep the infant in skin-to-skin contact with the mother during the early hours after birth. Skin-to-skin care heats the infant's entire body (peripheral and trunk) rather than just the trunk which is what happens under a radiant warmer (Christidis, Zotter, Rosegger, Engele, Kurz, & Kerbel, 2003). This avoids the possibility of chilling during the early hours as does delaying the infant bath.

  - Keep the mother and infant together (even at night).

- Do not allow the infant to cry.
- Immediately respond to any cries.

- There is a normal dip in blood glucose in the first one to four hours after birth.

  - Avoid giving sugar water by mouth, because it is metabolized rapidly, often before the infant can mount effective counter regulatory activities. This may cause rebound hypoglycemia.

  - Avoid testing blood sugar during this time with reagent strips (in asymptomatic, low-risk infants).

  - Provide unlimited access to the breast and ensure colostrum/milk transfer.

  - Delay the bath for at least 12 hours to avoid chilling the infant and to promote skin-to-skin contact.

- Feed expressed colostrum (not formula) if the infant is unable to latch or feeds poorly. Infants with risk factors for hypoglycemia should be fed frequently. Tozier (2013) demonstrated that glucose values of infants born to mothers with type one or gestational diabetes who were fed colostrum supplements were no different than those infants who received formula supplementation. Mothers expressed colostrum prenatally, during early labor, and/or following delivery, storing the colostrum in feeding syringes in the refrigerator or on ice. This colostrum was then used as a supplement in these at-risk infants following breastfeeding attempts during the early hours after birth. The recommendations from this study for infants of diabetic mothers include the following:

  - Feed the infant first, right after birth, before checking glucose values. The infant can be put to breast followed by expressed colostrum drops.

  - Obtain first glucose value by 90 minutes of age in an asymptomatic newborn.

  - Newborns have the opportunity to receive colostrum by spoon, syringe, or pipette in addition to breastfeeding to achieve glucose stabilization before any formula is given. Feed colostrum drops every couple of hours in addition to breastfeeding attempts.

  - As long as the newborn is asymptomatic, the initial glucose between 25 mg/dl and 40 mg/dl is acceptable.

  - The infant is then fed more colostrum drops, in addition to feeding at the breast with prolonged skin-to-skin contact.

- The second glucose value is checked one hour later, usually at two and a half to three hours of age.

- As long as the infant remains asymptomatic, the newborn has until four hours of age to achieve a blood glucose value of 40 mg/dl.

- If the infant remains asymptomatic, the glucose values are checked every three hours until 12 hours of age.

- The target values after the first four hours of life are 45 mg/dl until 24 hours of age and 50 mg/dl after 24 hours of age.

- The initial bath is delayed 12 hours.

Holmes (2013) provides recommendations that include direct breastfeeding attempts in the first three hours after birth for at-risk newborns with glucose levels between 28 and 39 mg/dl. If the feeding is ineffective or a repeat measure indicates persistent hypoglycemia, then 3-10 ml of expressed colostrum should be administered.

- The protein and fat in colostrum provide substrates for gluconeogenesis.

- Colostrum and breastmilk enhance ketogenesis.

- Colostrum increases gut motility and gastric emptying time, causing rapid absorption of nutrients.

- If the infant is unable to latch or effectively transfer colostrum, have the mother hand express colostrum into a spoon and spoon-feed it to the infant (using a pump often results in little to no colostrum being retrievable to feed to the infant, because it sticks to the sides of the bottle). If the mother is unable to express colostrum and has expressed colostrum prenatally, use this to spoon feed the infant.

Maternal request

Maternal request is a frequent reason seen in the hospital for supplementing infants with formula. Cultural factors are frequently attributed to this practice. However, DaMota et al. (2012) found in a sample of 97 English- and Spanish-speaking low-income mothers, that cultural factors were not mentioned as a reason for requesting formula supplementation. Lack of preparation for what the early postpartum period would be like actually determined mothers' request for the in-hospital use of infant formula. Mothers in this study described an event in the hospital that triggered the request for supplementation. Mothers overestimated the capabilities of a newborn and were not prepared for the frequency of feeding and waking in their newborn. Crying was interpreted as not enough milk, which called for using a bottle of formula. Unsettled behavior in the infant was thought to occur because the infant was not interested in breastfeeding or for the desire of infant formula. Many mothers thought their milk would come in immediately following delivery, that colostrum was insufficient for their infants, and that their infant would latch on easily and effectively the first time that they were put to breast. Some mothers were unaware that they would not have a large amount of milk immediately after birth, concluding that they did not have enough milk to satisfy the infant. Mothers did not realize that the small amounts of colostrum available during the early days were sufficient for their infants and used bottles of formula to assess how much milk their infants were lacking. Unmet infant expectations for their infant's behavior, perception that healthcare providers were unsupportive of breastfeeding, and the unexpected work of new parenting, led to the belief that infant formula was the solution to all of these problems. Some mothers who encountered breastfeeding problems requested infant formula rather than asking for help.

Given the unrealistic expectations of many mothers and the lack of understanding of the breastfeeding process, clinicians may be able to help reduce non-medically indicated supplementation of breastfed newborns by:

- Offering prenatal education and/or education immediately post delivery on the availability and amount of colostrum, that not all crying indicates hunger, and that many newborns do not feed effectively the first time they are put to breast.

- Assuring that mothers are taught techniques to maximize colostrum intake at each feeding, such as correct latch and alternate massage.

- Educating mothers regarding the frequency of newborn feeding, how to rest between feedings, and minimizing the number of visitors and interruptions.

- Intervening immediately to correct nipple pain or soreness.

- Explaining the capabilities and behavior of a newborn.

- Ascertaining how the mother interprets her infant's behavior.

- Assuring that mothers learn and can perform the basic skills necessary to recognize hunger cues, latch the infant with no pain, feed enough times each 24 hours, and understand how to maximize milk intake at each feeding.

Heinig, Banuelos, Goldbronn, and Kampp (2009) studied how infant behavior interpretation by mothers influenced formula supplementation of breastfed infants. Educating parents about infant sleep cycles, hunger cues, and newborn behaviors helped reduce unnecessary and excessive formula supplementation. Infant sleep cycles initially are 60 minutes long, with some infants waking with each cycle, every one to two hours. Mothers will often wish to supplement with formula when their infant displays fussiness or crying when put down after a breastfeeding. The mother picks up the infant and breastfeeds again, but the infant again fusses when put down. In this scenario check to make sure that the infant is actually swallowing colostrum/milk and have the mother use alternate massage (massage the breast during sucking pauses on each breast at each feeding) to assure milk/colostrum transfer. Infants in active sleep wake up easily when put down, because active sleep is a light sleep. When they are in quiet sleep, they are harder to wake up. Once assured that the infant has actually fed and swallowed colostrum/milk, have the mother wait 20 minutes after the feeding before putting baby down to assure that the infant is in a deeper sleep state and will not startle or wake.

Clinical Implications

Breastfeeding self-efficacy is the confidence a mother has in her ability to breastfeed her infant and how she will respond to breastfeeding difficulties (Dennis, 1999). Self-efficacy is a significant predictor of breastfeeding duration and exclusivity (Nichols, Schutte, Brown, Dennis, & Price, 2009). Infant behaviors also influence mothers' self-efficacy. Mothers associate specific infant behaviors with feeding satisfaction, which reinforces the mother's confidence in her ability to meet her infant's needs. Infants who demonstrate readiness to feed behaviors, ease of latching, and a strong sucking pattern are more likely to be exclusively breastfeeding at six weeks compared to infants who showed difficulty with these behaviors (Loke & Chan, 2013). Self-efficacy may be influenced by friends and relatives of the mother who provide positive support through encouragement to breastfeed and offer help to persevere in the face of problems. Friends and relatives who are discouraging in their interactions with a mother, who relate horror stories, describe pain, sleeplessness, frustration, or indifference to breastfeeding can override theoretical knowledge and science. A mother's decisions can be biased by anecdotal stories from friends and family about how they used formula and their baby turned out just fine. Stories told to a mother may be more influential than evidence-based information supplied by a healthcare provider. Stories are more vivid and easier to process than facts. Stories related about breastfeeding by healthcare providers may work to create a better connection between the mother and the clinician. Descriptions or imagery (rather than facts) that paint a story of how mothers can overcome obstacles may craft the desired response. This might help mothers place themselves in the situation being described to them of how they can overcome breastfeeding bumps in the road.

Community norms may also influence the propensity for many mothers to engage in infant formula supplementation. Neighborhood context or place-based contagion processes can influence health behaviors, as individuals model the behaviors of those around them. These processes shape the cultural norms of the neighborhood environment. Mothers rely on these norms when making decisions regarding engaging in specific health behaviors, such as breastfeeding and supplementation. Social norms that discourage breastfeeding have been shown to be prevalent in underprivileged environments where there are few role models to emulate breastfeeding behaviors (Bentley, Dee, & Jensen, 2003). The majority of low-income African-American mothers in one study had never seen someone in their neighborhood breastfeed and could not imagine themselves doing so in public (Kaufman, Deenadayalan, & Karpati, 2010). Burdette (2013) explored the relationship between neighborhood context and breastfeeding behaviors. Results of this study showed that residing in highly educated neighborhoods was associated with positive breastfeeding practices compared with low educational neighborhoods, but neighborhood racial and ethnic make-up was not related to breastfeeding practices. Individual and neighborhood context were shown to be independent predictors of breastfeeding behaviors. This suggested that individual approaches to desired health behaviors may be limited by barriers erected by neighborhood context. Clinicians desiring to improve exclusive breastfeeding rates may need to target interventions in specific neighborhoods and communities, such as improving hospital breastfeeding policies, engaging other neighborhood institutions to normalize breastfeeding, and providing exposure to more neighborhood role models.

Many mothers view breastfeeding as "perfect," but time-crunched mothers often settle for pragmatism rather than perfection. A rational approach to breastfeeding may contribute to why duration and exclusivity are not meeting their national targets. Context and experience may be more influential in breastfeeding than theoretical knowledge. A mother's health-related decisions are constantly adapting to changes in her environment. There may be a mismatch between idealism (six months of exclusive breastfeeding) and realism (immediate relief from nipple pain or obtaining more sleep by giving the infant formula bottles) (Hoddinott, Craig, Britten, & McInnes, 2012). When mothers are faced with breastfeeding problems or logistical difficulties in situations, such as returning to work, low milk supply, a fussy baby, pumping milk, caring for other children, or frequent feedings, the solution for some mothers is to supplement with formula, as it immediately relieves the tension between the ideal and the practical. Breastfeeding interventions that emphasize realistic short-term goals and present solutions to problems that are part of the mother's daily living experience might improve breastfeeding exclusivity.

Chapter 4. Medical Indications for Supplementation of Breastfed Infants

While much infant formula supplementation is not medically necessary, there are a number of infant and maternal factors that serve as indicators of the potential need for medically indicated supplementation. In 2009, the World Health Organization published a set of acceptable medical reasons for the use of breastmilk substitutes (Box 4.1) (World Health Organization, 2009).

Box 4.1. WHO Acceptable Reasons for Use of Breastmilk Substitutes

Infant Conditions

Infants who should not receive breastmilk or any other milk except specialized formula

Infants with classic galactosemia: a special galactose-free formula is needed.

Infants with maple syrup urine disease: a special formula free of leucine, isoleucine and valine is needed.

Infants with phenylketonuria: a special phenylalanine-free formula is needed (breastfeeding is possible, under careful monitoring).

Infants for whom breastmilk remains the best feeding option, but who may need other food in addition to breastmilk for a limited period

Infants born weighing less than 1500 g (very low birth weight).

Infants born at less than 32 weeks of gestational age (very preterm).

Newborn infants who are at risk of hypoglycemia by virtue of impaired metabolic adaptation or increased glucose demand (such as those who are preterm, small for gestational age or who have experienced significant intrapartum hypoxic/ischaemic stress, those who are ill and those whose mothers are diabetic) (5) if their blood sugar fails to respond to optimal breastfeeding or breastmilk feeding.

Maternal Conditions

Maternal conditions that may justify permanent avoidance of breastfeeding

HIV infection1: if replacement feeding is acceptable, feasible, affordable, sustainable and safe

Maternal conditions that may justify temporary avoidance of breastfeeding

Severe illness that prevents a mother from caring for her infant, for

Herpes simplex virus type 1 (HSV-1): direct contact between lesions on the mother's breasts and the infant's mouth should be avoided until all active lesions have resolved.

Maternal medication:

- sedating psychotherapeutic drugs, anti-epileptic drugs and opioids and their combinations may cause side effects such as drowsiness and respiratory depression and are better avoided if a safer alternative is available

- radioactive iodine-131 is better avoided given that safer alternatives are available - a mother can resume breastfeeding about two months after receiving this substance

- excessive use of topical iodine or iodophors (e.g., povidone-iodine), especially on open wounds or mucous membranes, can result in thyroid suppression or electrolyte abnormalities in the breastfed infant and should be avoided

- cytotoxic chemotherapy requires that a mother stops breastfeeding during therapy

Source: World Health Organization. (2009). *Acceptable medical reasons for use of breast-milk substitutes.* Geneva, Switzerland. http://whqlibdoc.who.int/hq/2009/ WHO_FCH_CAH_09.01_eng.pdf Used with permission.

The Academy of Breastfeeding Medicine developed an evidence-based supplementation protocol with indications for supplementation where breastfeeding is not possible, as well as a set of indications for possible supplementation (Box 4.2) (Academy of Breastfeeding Medicine, 2009).

Prior to supplementation, a thorough breastfeeding assessment and evaluation of the mother and infant should be conducted, including a direct observation of a feeding at the breast. Also included should be an evaluation of the maternal milk supply; a labor, delivery, and feeding history; an evaluation of the infant's positioning, latch, suck, and swallow; and an assessment of the infant's overall condition. In order to best assist new mothers, many clinicians have found it helpful to have scripts available as a means of immediately addressing supplementation situations. Such scripts may be especially beneficial when the supplementation has been requested by the mother rather than for an actual medical indication. Scripting can be an effective communication tool, allowing clinicians to face challenging situations with confidence and consistency. Sincere, well-scripted phrases can set the stage for meaningful teaching opportunities and help mothers

Box 4.2. Academy of Breastfeeding Medicine Indications for Supplementation of the Breastfed Infant

Indications for supplementation of healthy term infants where breastfeeding is not possible

1. Separation

- Maternal illness resulting in separation of infant and mother (e.g., shock or psychosis)
- Mother not at the same hospital

2. Infant with inborn error of metabolism (e.g., galactosemia)

3. Infant who is unable to feed at the breast (e.g., congenital malformation, illness)

4. Maternal medications (those contraindicated in breastfeeding)

Possible indications for supplementation of term healthy infants

1. Infant indications

- Asymptomatic hypoglycemia documented by laboratory blood glucose measurement (not bedside screening methods) that is unresponsive to appropriate frequent breastfeeding. Symptomatic infants should be treated with intravenous glucose. (See ABM Hypoglycemia Protocol for more details.)
- Clinical and laboratory evidence of significant dehydration (e.g., 10% weight loss, high sodium, poor feeding, lethargy, etc.) that is not improved after skilled assessment and proper management of breastfeeding
- Weight loss of 8-10% accompanied by delayed lactogenesis II (day five [120 hours] or later)
- Delayed bowel movements or continued meconium stools on day five (120 hours)
- Insufficient intake despite an adequate milk supply (poor milk transfer)
- Hyperbilirubinemia
  - i. "Neonatal" jaundice associated with starvation where breastmilk intake is poor despite appropriate intervention (please see ABM Jaundice in the Breastfed Infant Protocol)
  - ii. Breastmilk jaundice when levels reach 20-25 mg/dl (mol/L) in an otherwise thriving infant and where a diagnostic and/or therapeutic interruption of breastfeeding may be helpful
- When macronutrient supplementation is indicated

2. Maternal indications

- Delayed lactogenesis II (day three to five or later [72–120 hours] and inadequate intake by the infant

  - Retained placenta (lactogenesis probably will occur after placental fragments are removed)

  - Sheehan's syndrome (postpartum hemorrhage followed by absence of lactogenesis)

  - Primary glandular insufficiency, occurs in less than 5% of women (primary lactation failure), as evidenced by poor breast growth during pregnancy and minimal indications of lactogenesis

- Breast pathology or prior breast surgery resulting in poor milk production

- Intolerable pain during feedings unrelieved by interventions

Source: Academy of Breastfeeding Medicine. (2009).Hospital guidelines for the use of supplementary feedings in the healthy term breastfed neonate. Clinical Protocol #3. Revised 2009. *Breastfeeding Medicine.* 4,175-182. Used with permission.

through anxious or frustrating situations (Table 4.1). A useful approach to maternal request for supplementation includes the HEART approach (Garrison, Byrne, & Moore, 2009):

- **H**ear your patient. Look at her and listen carefully to what she is saying or describing. Check to make sure you are interpreting the exchange correctly—"I think I hear you saying that…" Clarifying her problem can help devise a more rapid and accurate approach to the reason she wants to supplement the infant.

- **E**mpathize with her concern. This lets her know that you are taking her concerns seriously. "I can understand how this makes you feel…" or "Many mothers have told me the same thing you are describing, so you are not alone!"

- **A**pologize if she has not received the help that she needs. Help her understand that you are also concerned about the issue. "I am sorry that this is such a frustrating experience for you."

- **R**espond. "Let's take a look at how baby is feeding…" or "Let me see what I can do to help."

- **T**hank. "It was my pleasure to help you with this issue." Positive reinforcement for her request for help can encourage the mother to continue to ask for help, not just in the hospital, but also following discharge. Some mothers are hesitant to ask for help, so it is beneficial to assure the mother that there is plenty of help available to her.

Table 4.1. Scripting Examples

Maternal concern	Possible script	Intervention
"I don't have enough milk."	Many mothers worry about this. What makes you think you don't have enough milk?	Feeding observation of baby at breast. Assess for colostrum/milk transfer. Review stages of lactation, appearance and quantity of colostrum, colostrum/milk intake per feeding.
"My baby is still hungry and not satisfied after a feeding."	Why do feel your baby is not getting enough colostrum/milk?	Feeding observation to check for swallowing. Use breast compressions on each breast at each feeding to increase intake.
"My baby wakes up and cries as soon as I put him down after a feeding."	Sometimes babies are in a light sleep state after a feeding and wake easily when put down.	Assure adequate milk transfer. Have mother hold baby for 20 minutes following feedings before putting him down.
"My baby is sleepy and does not wake to feed."	Let's look at how to figure out the best time to feed your baby.	Rather than using the clock to determine when to feed the infant, use behavioral or readiness feeding cues (rapid eye movements under the eyelids, hand-to-mouth movements, sucking movements of the mouth, body movements, and small sounds.

"My baby fights at the breast or pushes away from the breast."	This can be really frustrating. Let's check to see if we can better position baby.	Try laid back or ventral positioning.
"My nipples are too sore to breastfeed."	I'm sorry to hear that. Let's see what we can do to make it better.	Feeding observation, assuring that the infant's mouth is open wide at a 160-degree angle. If too painful at breast, hand express colostrum/milk and feed to baby.
"My baby feeds too frequently."	Some babies cluster or bunch their feedings into short periods of time. Your baby's stomach is very small and colostrum/milk is digested very rapidly.	Assess feedings for milk transfer. Use breast compressions when feeding to assure maximum colostrum/milk intake. Reassure mother that clustered or bunched feedings are common and not an indication for formula supplementation.
"I was fed formula and I am OK or I fed my first and/or subsequent babies formula and he/they are OK."	While you were fed formula or your other children were fed formula, it is not the same as breastmilk. I am happy to help you get off to a good start to avoid having to supplement.	Ask why she wants to supplement. Review the differences between formula and breastmilk. Make each breastfeeding session a positive experience.

Many mothers will request formula supplementation when they feel that their baby is not getting enough colostrum or milk at the breast. They may be frustrated or fatigued due to frequent and/or ineffective feedings. Infant behaviors are usually described that have caused the mother to interpret them as the baby not receiving enough milk. Fussy, unsettled behavior, especially following a feeding at breast may trigger the request for formula supplementation. Clinicians may find that a loosely scripted approach such as the one in Box 4.3 will help decrease or eliminate the actual need to supplement. The goals are to identify the mother's actual concern, interpret the infant's behavior, assess the feeding to determine if the infant is transferring colostrum or milk, and teach the mother signs of milk transfer and adequate feeds. This approach looks to help decrease the perceived need to supplement.

To help both clinicians and parents understand the possible undesirable outcomes of supplementing breastfed infants with formula, some hospitals use a consent form as a teaching tool. These forms generally describe the potential ramifications of formula supplementation and ask that the mother sign to indicate she understands the potential outcomes. Many hospitals also have a policy that requires a lactation consultant visit to the mother at the next breastfeed following bottle supplementation to assure that the infant can still feed from the breast. Links to sample forms can be found in the Resources section at the end of this book.

Because unnecessary formula supplementation can be such a problem, some hospitals have taken steps to help clinicians reduce this practice and track supplementation patterns. Infant formula bottles may be stored in a special or locked cabinet where nurses must sign out each bottle, recording the name of the patient, why the bottle is being given, and the name of the nurse or clinician who obtains the bottle. Other hospitals have put formula bottles in their medication distribution system, such as a Pyxis system. This demonstrates that formula supplementation is to be used in a manner similar to medication, that is, only when medically necessary. This system can track formula usage and serve to indicate where additional staff education may be necessary.

Some maternity unit staff distribute supplemental formula to breastfeeding patients, justifying such practices by telling patients that they were fed formula or that they fed their own children formula and they all turned out just fine. This type of rationalization may be engaged in to help protect clinicians from feeling bad about their own past behaviors, that somehow they engaged in less-than-optimal parenting behaviors, or in an attempt to protect mothers from feeling "guilty" if they supplement with formula. However, we do not see clinicians on a cardiac unit telling patients that they eat fast food double cheeseburgers and they feel fine, so it is OK for the patient to eat this too. No coupons are given out for fast food when heart attack patients are discharged. This situation is ultimately cognitive dissonance: to not give out formula would be to admit that something clinicians have been doing for up to decades is wrong—that the clinician has been doing something wrong for decades. One's very identity as a

Box 4.3. Scripting and Teaching for Maternal Requested Supplementation

- "You are saying that the baby is not satisfied after a feeding and that you don't think he is getting enough milk at the breast. Let's look at a feeding to see what he is doing."
  - Review positioning, latch, suck, and swallow. Determine if the baby is swallowing milk. Correct positioning and latch if necessary. Assure that the mother knows the signs of swallowing.
  - Ask the mother to verbalize when the baby is swallowing colostrum/milk.
  - Have the mother use breast compression/alternate massage on each breast at each feeding to maximize milk transfer.
- "Let's review how to know that the baby is getting enough." Teaching points can include:
  - Your baby's stomach capacity is very small at first and colostrum/milk is digested much faster than formula.
  - Baby may take in only a quarter to half an ounce at each breastfeeding during the first day or two. This gradually increases as he gets older.
  - Baby may show lots more interest in feeding on day two and three, especially at night! Some nurses call feeding patterns on day two the "all day buffet!" Babies may also cluster or bunch their feedings in the late afternoon and early evening such that they feed every hour or so for a period of time. These feeding patterns do not mean that he isn't getting enough milk or that there is something wrong with your milk supply.
  - Feeding frequently during these times and making sure that baby is swallowing gets lots of disease-fighting colostrum and milk into baby and helps increase your milk supply.
  - "It must seem that baby is always wanting to feed and that he does not sleep for very long."
    - ◆ In the early days, babies cycle sleep in one hour time periods. Sometimes babies wake each time they cycle into a lighter sleep state.
    - ◆ If your baby falls asleep in your arms after breastfeeding and will no longer suck and swallow when you compress the breast, then wait 20 minutes before putting him down in the bassinette.

- "Let's review the signs that the baby is getting enough."
  - No longer sucking and swallowing when mothers do breast compressions.
  - Diaper count of one wet diaper on day one, two wet diapers on day two, three wet diapers on day three; one meconium stooling on day one, two meconium stools on day two, transitioning from meconium to greenish stools on day three, and no uric acid crystals after day three.
  - If baby is being weighed pre- and post-feeds, intake should be 2-10 ml per feed in the first 24 hours, 5-15 ml per feed from 24-48 hours, 15-30 ml per feed from 48-72 hours, and 30-60 ml per feed from 72-96 hours.
  - Baby should lose between five to eight percent of birth weight depending on urine and stooling output.
- "While giving baby bottles of formula may make him sleep, it may interfere with feeding at the breast and your milk production. Giving baby formula during this time can interfere with the programming of the immune system."
  - Formula supplements can delay the maturation of the gut (intestine) and increase the chances of bowel infections, allergies, obesity, diabetes, and other diseases and conditions.
  - Most of the immune system lives in the gut. Breastmilk directs how beneficial bacteria are lured to the gut and bad bacteria are routed into the diaper.
  - Formula is made from cow's milk, and even small amounts can sensitize the baby to allergy and diabetes.
  - Formula decreases the amount of breastmilk the baby gets and can decrease baby's protection from disease.
  - Artificial nipples on bottles can change the way baby sucks, increasing the chances of sore nipples and problems with how the baby will feed at the breast.
  - Giving baby a bottle of formula after breastfeeding is not a way to determine how much milk baby did or did not get from the breast.
  - Formula supplements may cause the baby to be less interested in feeding at the breast.

competent nurse or a doctor seems to be called into question. When changing policies or working to decrease unnecessary formula supplementation, this needs to be acknowledged and respected. Other contributors to unnecessary formula supplementation include:

- Clinicians fear breastfed infants will develop hypoglycemia and supplement routinely to prevent this from happening on their shift or to their patients.

- Clinicians may fear omission more than commission and give formula supplements. They would rather give a bottle than miss something.

- Clinicians may have experienced a bad outcome in a previous patient, therefore supplementing all babies to make sure it does not happen again.

- Empathy for a tired mother may motivate some clinicians to suggest formula supplementation.

- Formula supplementation may be a quicker solution to breastfeeding issues, may be used when staff is frustrated or fatigued, or may be resorted to when clinicians do not know how to help a mother.

It may help staff reduce unnecessary formula supplementation if they document the reasons they give formula. The act of confronting the issue may help change behaviors and find solutions. Not all hospitals have lactation consultants (LC) on staff, or if they do, there may not be enough lactation consultants to meet patient census and acuity. Optimal lactation consultant-to-patient ratios are 1.3 LCs per 1,000 births in a Level I hospital, 1.6 LCs per 1,000 births in a Level II hospital, and 1.9 LCs per 1,000 births in a Level III hospital (United States Lactation Consultant Association, 2010). Utilization of International Board Certified Lactation Consultants (IBCLC) has been shown to improve exclusive breastfeeding rates, both in hospital (Castrucci, Hoover, Lim, & Maus, 2006) and following discharge (Bonuck, Stuebe, Barnett, Labbok, Fletcher, & Bernstein, 2014). Hospitals without 24/7 LC coverage may wish to provide advanced training to some of their nurses to act as lactation resource nurses on each shift to assure patient access to lactation care that meets their needs.

Helping hospitals to achieve higher exclusive breastfeeding rates and to lower the amount of formula supplementation can be quite a challenge. Clinicians may wish to utilize a change model known as Quality Improvement (QI) and ask the hospital QI department to convene a multi-disciplinary committee or task force to address practice problems on the maternity unit (Cadwell, 1997). Through the use of QI tools, improvement in practices proceed to define the problem, determine what should be happening versus what **is** happening, and what can be done to achieve current, evidence-based practice. Actions and interventions are data-driven and evidence-based such that one person or the notion that "we have always done it this way" cannot impede practice improvement. Data-driven activities help assure unbiased change. Evidence-based medically indicated supplementation for breastfed infants is a goal that is perfectly suited for a QI project. The New York State Department of Health designed an 18-month breastfeeding quality improvement in hospitals project to help increase rates of exclusive breastfeeding during the birth, hospitalization, and beyond (FitzPatrick, Dennison, Welge, Hisgen, Boyce, & Waniewski, 2013). In their Change Package, they recommended seven supporting strategies to reduce unnecessary formula supplementation:

- Place a sign in infant's bassinet stating that the infant is breastfeeding and that no bottle feeding of any type should be offered.

- Provide no supplemental water, glucose, or formula to breastfeeding infants unless specified by a written physician order for a clinical condition or by the mother's documented and informed request.

- Prior to non-medically indicated supplementation of breastfed infants (i.e., mother's request), mothers are informed of the risks of supplementation to the establishment and success of breastfeeding. The mother's request and discussion of the risks are documented in the medical record.

- Utilize an alternative feeding method, such as a cup (recommended), dropper, or syringe, to maintain mother-infant breastfeeding skills when supplementation is medically indicated.

- Do NOT place bottles in a breastfeeding infant's bassinet.

- Document infant feeding in the medical record each shift.

- Institute inventory controls for formula similar to other foods, medications, and/or supplies (e.g., include formula in automated dispensing and distribution systems).

Chapter 5. What, How, and How Much to Supplement

What to supplement

Once the recommendation for medically-indicated supplementation is made, the question then becomes what type of supplement should be used? A list of supplemental feeding types in preferential order can be found in Table 5.1.

Table 5.1. Supplemental Feeding Types in Preferential Order

- Fresh expressed mother's own colostrum/milk
- Refrigerated mother's own milk
- Frozen and thawed mother's own milk
- Fortified (if necessary) mother's own milk for preterm infants
- Pasteurized banked donor human milk
- Hypoallergenic (hydrolyzed) infant formula
- Elemental Infant formula
- Cow's-milk-based infant formula
- Soy Infant formula
- Water

Fresh, expressed mother's own milk is always preferable to use as a supplement (American Academy of Pediatrics, 2012) unless very rare conditions or situations temporarily or permanently preclude its use. Given that some babies may require supplementation soon after birth, the practice of prenatal colostrum expression has been used to have a ready supply of colostrum available in the immediate postpartum period. The practice of antenatal breast expression can be effective as a means of avoiding the use of infant formula if supplementation should be required for babies of diabetic mothers or other infants who are known prenatally to be at risk for hypoglycemia or early feeding problems. Other potential indications for the prenatal expression of colostrum include infants who have been diagnosed prenatally with cleft palate or a neurologic or cardiac condition, a family history of allergy to cow's milk, a history of maternal low milk supply, or any other condition in the infant that would present challenges to early breastfeeding success. However, large, credible randomized controlled trials of this practice have not been conducted (Chapman, Pincomb, & Harris, 2013). Small studies of prenatal colostrum expression have yielded positive results, with a reduced reliance on infant formula as a supplement and a more rapid arrival at exclusive breastfeeding (Gurneesh & Ellora, 2009; Singh, Chouhan, & Sidhu, 2009).

Prenatal colostrum expression was described by mothers in a study by Brisbane and Giglia (2013) as bolstering their confidence in being able to breastfeed. Visualizing the expressed colostrum provided reassurance that the breasts were functioning normally. Mothers mentioned the feeling of security in knowing that they had a ready supply of breastmilk for use in case there were early feeding problems. Mastery of colostrum expression and confirmation of the presence of colostrum served to increase the mothers' self-efficacy that they would be able to carry out the steps necessary to successfully breastfeed their baby. The antenatal expression of colostrum allowed the mothers to become competent and familiar with breastmilk expression by hand. This is a skill that is helpful for all new breastfeeding mothers and one that is assessed if a hospital is seeking the Baby Friendly designation. Having a supply of expressed colostrum immediately available can help reduce maternal stress over milk supply, especially when there is a known risk factor for the possibility of medically indicated supplementation.

Some concern has been advanced regarding the possibility of inducing contractions or premature labor by the nipple stimulation experienced when expressing colostrum prenatally. Breastfeeding during pregnancy has not been proven to be unsafe nor has antenatal colostrum expression, given the multitude of factors, other than oxytocin release, that predispose or induce premature labor. Forster et al. (2011) showed that cardiotocographs performed after antenatal colostrum expression showed no signs of any fetal compromise. Barring known risk factors, pregnant breastfeeding mothers have not been found to be at an increased risk for preterm labor (Moscone & Moore, 1993). Mothers with the following conditions should not express colostrum prenatally: have a history of threatened or actual premature labor, are currently having problems with threatened premature labor and are taking medication to prevent it, have cervical insufficiency, have a cervical cerclage (stitches in the cervix to hold it closed), are carrying twins or higher order multiples, or experience contractions when expressing colostrum. Due to the clear benefits of early colostrum feedings and the potential hazardous effects of early formula supplementation, antenatal colostrum expression should outweigh the unsupported risks of prenatal colostrum expression education (Cox, 2010). However, each mother needs to consider this in relation to her own situation and her potential risks and benefits. Diabetic mothers may wish to express colostrum prenatally, freeze it, and bring it to the hospital in case their infant requires supplementation (Cox, 2006). This may be especially important since delayed lactogenesis II is common in diabetic mothers. Mothers can begin expressing colostrum daily for three to five minutes on each breast by drawing it into a 1 ml or 3 ml syringe at 37 weeks, as long as they experience no uterine cramping.

The potential risks and benefits of supplementation must be considered within the overall goal of preserving breastfeeding (Academy of Breastfeeding Medicine, 2009). Each type of supplement (Table 5.2) should be considered in terms of its potential to provide appropriate nutrition, protect the maternal milk supply, and avoid feeding-related morbidities (Wight, 2001).

How Much to Supplement

The stomach of a newborn infant is small and somewhat noncompliant. This means that the stomach does not easily relax to accommodate a feeding during the early hours after birth. During the next three days of life, a reduction in gastric tone and an increase in compliance allow the stomach to accept increasing volumes of milk per feeding (Zangen, Di Lorenzo, Zangen, Mertz, Schwankovsky, & Hyman, 2001). Clinically, this change is seen as infants ingesting very small volumes of milk and regurgitating milk or formula if they are coaxed to swallow in excess of what their stomachs can physiologically accommodate.

There is a difference between the physiological and anatomical capacity of the newborn stomach. The physiological capacity is what an infant can comfortably ingest at a feeding (feeding volume as determined by pre- and post-feed weights), whereas the anatomical capacity is what the stomach will hold at its maximum fullness (such as determined on autopsy or when distress occurs). Various authors using different methods and calculations have provided estimates of the volume of the newborn stomach. Physiological capacity (Scammon & Doyle, 1920) is considerably less than anatomical capacity during the early days. Physiological and anatomical stomach capacities begin to approximate each other around four days of age. The actual size of the newborn stomach has received little attention, especially in regards to the volume of what a "normal" feeding should be. Widstrom et al. (1988) studied gastric aspirates in newborns immediately after birth, showing gastric contents of 0-11 ml. They suggested that the fetus typically drinks about 10 ml portions of amniotic fluid, which are gradually emptied from the stomach.

Table 5.2. Supplement Comparison

Supplement	Calories per ounce	Allergic potential	Effect on milk production	Effect on bilirubin levels	Effect on blood sugar	Effect on infant gut
Expressed mother's milk	18 colostrum 20 or more mature	None	Increases	Normal	Stabilizes and increases	Protects and programs the gut immune system; accelerates gut closure
Cow's-milk-based formula	20	High	Decreases	Lowers	Increases	Adversely alters gut integrity; delays gut closure
Soy formula	20	Medium to high	Decreases	Lowers	Increases	Adversely alters gut integrity
Hydrolyzed formula	20	Low	Decreases	Lowers	Increases	Adversely alters gut integrity
Sterile water	0	None	Decreases	Increases	None	None
D_5W	6	None	Decreases	Increases	Bounces	None

Source: Adapted from Walker, M. (2014). *Breastfeeding management for the clinician: using the evidence.* Burlington, MA, Jones & Bartlett Learning.

Using real-time ultrasound imaging, Nagata, Koyanagi, Fukushima, Akazawa, and Nakano (1994) calculated fetal stomach volume at 38 weeks to be approximately 9.9 ml, whereas Sase et al. (2005) using ultrasound calculated newborn stomach volumes at approximately 10 ml. Naveed, Manjunath, and Sreenivas (1992) calculated the anatomical stomach capacity at autopsy of 100 perinatal stillbirths and 37 deaths occurring in the first week. They found that larger infants had a greater anatomical stomach capacity than smaller infants. An infant over 5.5 lb (2,500 g) was shown to have an anatomical capacity of 18-21 ml. Hata et al. (2010) used three-dimensional ultrasound to study the volume of the fetal stomach. They reported that the fetal gastric volume calculated by 2-D ultrasound is about one third smaller than the maximum volume using 3-D ultrasound. These authors found that at 36 weeks, the maximum volume of the fetal stomach was almost 14 ml. The functional capacity was somewhat less. Goldstein et al. (1987) measured fetal stomach size by ultrasound over the course of the pregnancy. Mathematical calculations from their data yield a stomach size at near term of 12 ml. Kernesiuk, Levchik, and Vilkova (1997) measured stomach dimensions in term infants at autopsy and reported a stomach capacity of 15 ml. Zangen et al. (2001) estimated that newborn stomach capacity is between 15 ml and 20 ml, as intake of 30 ml causes distress. Bergman (2013) calculated that a newborn infant's stomach capacity is approximately 20 ml. These studies offer a range of newborn stomach volumes from 9.9 ml to 21 ml.

One study actually measured the intake of colostrum at feedings during the first 24 hours in 90 healthy newborn infants. Using a highly sensitive scale, intake was measured during eight-hour periods of time. The amount of colostrum ingested was evaluated in 307 feedings with 3.4 ± 1 feedings recorded per eight-hour observation period. Mean gain per feeding was 1.5 ± 1.1 g. The volume of milk ingested by newborn infants during the first 24 hours was estimated at 15 ± 11 g (Santoro, Martinez, Ricco, & Jorge, 2010).

While newborn stomach volume calculations give the clinician an idea of the size of the stomach, infants may not necessarily have a milk intake that equals their anatomic stomach volume each time they feed, especially in the first day after birth.

Communicating the concept of the small stomach size and the need for small feedings and avoidance of large formula supplements during the early days led to the concept of a visual aid to illustrate the small size of the newborn stomach (Spangler, Randenberg, Brenner, & Howett, 2008). Objects such as marbles, ping-pong balls, and eggs serve to illustrate the approximate breastmilk intake of infants at various ages and help parents and clinicians understand that encouraging infants to take volumes beyond their physiological capacity may be detrimental. The anatomical and physiological capacities of the newborn stomach vary widely and depend on gestational age and feeding history. There is really no single visual aid, such as a walnut, that accurately reflects the exact volume a specific infant can safely consume. Many clinicians use a teaspoon to represent an average feeding volume on day one because 5 ml is within the range of intakes of normal term breastfed infants.

Human milk is easily and rapidly digested. The mean gastric half-emptying time for formula is 65 minutes (range, 27-98 minutes), whereas the mean gastric half-emptying time for breastmilk is 47 minutes (range, 16-86 minutes) (Lambrecht, Robberecht, Deschynkel, & Afschrift, 1988; Van den Driessche, Peeters, Marien, Ghoos, Devileger, & Veerman-Wauters, 1999). Thus breastfed infants can be hungry sooner than two or three hours after a feeding. Routine or capricious supplementation of a breastfed infant with water or formula after nursing is not supported by the data.

The amount of supplement to be provided also depends on the situation. Wight (2006) recommended 3-5 ml/kg of expressed breastmilk or breastmilk substitute. This volume is based on normal volumes of colostrum, the average size of the infant's stomach, and average volumes of milk typically ingested by newborns. If an infant needed an entire feeding supplemented, this amount may vary based on the infant's health status, weight, and feeding goals. For late preterm infants, Stellwagen, Hubbard, and Wolf (2007) recommend feeding volumes of 5-10 ml every two to three hours on day one, 10-20 ml on day two, and 20-30 ml on day three.

The volume of colostrum an infant ingests each day during the hospital stay is much lower than the 60 ml that is present in the ready-to-feed infant formula bottles used in the hospital. These bottles can give the appearance that a newborn infant should be consuming much more volume than his stomach can handle. Use of formula bottles could compel clinicians and mothers to persist in coaxing an infant to consume much more supplement than is physiologically appropriate. To avoid the appearance of providing much more supplement than is necessary, clinicians could prepare 10 ml aliquots of formula in a syringe or small medicine cup for supplementation, modeling appropriate formula amounts should medically indicated formula supplementation be necessary.

How to Supplement

There are several devices or implements available for supplementing a breastfed infant. Healthcare providers are not in agreement regarding practice and beliefs surrounding supplementation methods (Al-Sahab, Feldman, Macpherson, Ohlsson, & Tamim, 2010). Clinicians frequently recommend that the supplement be delivered by bottle, because it presents a well-known, rapid, and easy way to feed an infant. However, the sucking action on an artificial nipple is not the same as suckling from the breast. Huang, Gau, Huang, and Lee (2009) demonstrated that full-term infants supplemented with bottles displayed more negative sucking behavior during attempts to latch to the breast and that mothers who used bottles to supplement breastfeeding had a lower perception of milk supply up to four weeks postpartum. Perioral muscle function differs between bottle-feeding and breastfeeding (Inoue, Sakashita, & Kamegai, 1995). Artificial nipples that require mostly suction rather than mostly compression can contribute to reduced masseter muscle activity as the muscle adjusts to bottle-feeding (Sakashita, Kamegai, & Inoue, 1996). Geddes et al. (2012) conducted a study on the Calma (Medela, Inc.) nipple that requires only suction (vacuum) to remove milk from the bottle. Compression on this nipple will not remove milk. A minimum vacuum of -29 mm Hg was required to initiate milk flow. The mean peak vacuum applied during feeding with this nipple was significantly weaker than the peak vacuum of a baby who is feeding at breast (-67 compared with -122 mm Hg). The baseline vacuum applied to this nipple was also weaker than that which an infant applies at breast (-12 compared with -31 mm Hg). Segami, Mizuno, Taki, and Itabashi (2013) measured the intraoral pressure of infants feeding with the Calma nipple (Medela, Inc.), showing that baseline vacuum (that necessary to hold the nipple in the mouth) ranged from -51mm Hg to -10 mm Hg compared with the baseline vacuum in breastfeeding infants, which ranged from -80 mm Hg to -12 mm Hg. Peak pressure during breastfeeding in this study ranged from -255.4 to -74.6 mm Hg, and for feeding on the artificial nipple, the peak pressure ranged from -189 mm Hg to -50.8 mm Hg. Both peak pressure and baseline pressure were significantly smaller on the artificial nipple. Baseline vacuum elongates and positions the human nipple in the mouth and keeps it there, making sure that vacuum is not lost following each suck. These reduced vacuums are of concern if an infant who was fed with this nipple applied the same reduced vacuums to the breast and was unable to sufficiently draw in, elongate, and hold the nipple in place, and generated vacuum too low for milk removal. Buccinator muscles are recruited to compensate for altered tongue function during bottle-feeding. Changes in tongue function alter and weaken other muscles, such as the styloglossus and palatoglossus, used during sucking and swallowing. This change in oral muscle function may contribute to an infant experiencing difficulty in transitioning to the breast after being bottle-fed (Ferrante, Silvestri, & Montinaro, 2006). There can be significant differences between bottle feeding and breastfeeding in terms of swallowing and the stability of the suck-swallow-breathe cycle (Goldfield, Richardson, Lee, & Margetts, 2006). Mizuno and Ueda (2006) reported that sucking pressures for nutritive and non-nutritive sucking are exactly the opposite when comparing breastfeeding and sucking on an artificial nipple. Random, frequent, and uncoordinated swallowing seen with some bottle-feeding systems can contribute to desaturation, poor intake, and a delay in breastfeeding skill acquisition.

If supplementation is done by bottle, choice of an artificial nipple can be problematic. Nipple flow rates, shapes, and the necessary sucking mechanics are not standardized, many nipples are too stiff for an infant with a weak suck, some have rapid flow rates that compromise ventilation, and none fit the anatomical shape of an infant's oral structures. The mechanics of sucking on specific artificial nipples have been sparsely studied (Fadavi, Punwani, Jain, & Vidyasagar, 1997; Goldfield et al., 2006), and care must be taken in interpreting the results, because nipple parameters (material, deflection, flow rates, types of openings, and extension capabilities) are changed frequently by manufacturers. Aizawa, Mizuno, and Tamura (2010) demonstrated that the angle of mouth opening on the breast was double that of infants feeding from a standard size artificial nipple. A partially closed mouth configuration (as often seen with artificial nipples) on the breast may result in nipple pain, damage, and reduced milk intake.

When choosing an artificial nipple for a breastfed infant, consider the following. The artificial nipple should have a soft nipple (silicone rather than latex) that can be slightly elongated and deflected upward, mimicking the shape changes of the human nipple/areola. The human nipple is not stationary during breastfeeding and has a mean movement of 4.0 ± 1.3 mm during infant sucking (Jacobs, Dickinson, Hart, Doherty, & Faulkner, 2007). If the strength required to alter the artificial nipple shape is beyond the infant's capacity, the tongue may be forced down, reinforcing an incorrect swallow pattern (Ferrante et al., 2006).

The length of the artificial nipple must also be considered. Jacobs et al. (2007) found on ultrasound scans that the tip of the human nipple was usually not drawn into the mouth to a point where it rested directly under the junction of the hard and soft palates, but was positioned approximately 5 mm in front of this spot. The artificial nipple should not be so long that it causes the infant to gag. Shorter, softer, more mobile nipples may result in a supplementation experience that may not compromise too severely the transition to feeding at the breast.

Artificial nipples are typically less elastic than the human nipple, may elongate only minimally (Nowak, Smith, & Erenberg, 1994), may have varying flow rates (Mathew, 1988, 1990) which may or may not be appropriate for an individual infant, and may deliver milk using only vacuum or only compression rather than both. Pados, Estrem, Nix, Park, and Thoyre (2013) studied the flow rates (ml/minute) in 10 each of 15 types of nipples (Table 5.3).

The nipples that were advertised as "slow flow" all provided a different flow rate. The study demonstrated that the names of the nipples did not accurately describe the milk flow rates that could be expected. Clinicians may wish to consider the use of slower flowing nipples if supplementation is to be provided by bottle. Flow rates that are too fast for a breastfed infant could encourage the baby to be a reactive feeder rather than a proactive one. Babies who react to fast flow rates by using their tongue to slow the fluid flowing from the nipple, either by thrusting the tongue tip forward or bunching the tongue in the back, are engaging in oral mechanics that will not transfer milk from the breast. Breastfeeding is proactive in that the baby must engage in the extrusion reflex, pull in the nipple and part of the areola to form a teat, hold it in place, activate the tongue to remove milk from the breast, and exert sufficient vacuum to facilitate milk flow. Bottle-feeding can extinguish these behaviors in some infants, making supplementation by bottle a less than optimal choice.

The "orthodontic" type of nipple may eliminate the central grooving of the tongue (Wolf & Glass, 1992). Random, frequent, and uncoordinated swallowing seen with some bottle systems can provoke oxygen desaturation, poor intake, and a delay in breastfeeding skill acquisition, especially in a compromised infant. If a bottle is used, paced feedings may avoid fatigue and desaturation in less mature infants. Muscles of mastication along with jaw development may be temporarily affected with short-term supplementation or permanently changed with long-term bottle use.

The shape of the artificial nipple influences the infant's mouth conformation. Hoover (1996) found that pain-free breastfeeding occurred when the infant's mouth was open to an angle of 130-160 degrees (as measured at the corner of the mouth). Aizawa et al. (2010) found that infants only open their mouth to a 60-degree angle on conventional or standard narrow nipples. Infant mouth opening was shown to be 140 degrees on the Calma (Medela, Inc.) nipple (Segami et al., 2013). Peterson

Table 5.3. Flow Rates From Various Artificial Nipple Units

Brand	Flow rate (ml/minute)	Comments
Enfamil standard	18.92	
slow flow	14.68	
cross cut	2.10	
Similac standard	6.61	
slow flow	7.49	
premature	13.86	
Bionix Level 1	6.29	5 levels of flow; Level 1 provided slower flow than the others, but Levels 2-5 were not significantly different from one another
Dr. Brown's preemie	7.28	
Level 1	9.21	
Level 2	14.96	
Medela Calma	24.74	Provided the fastest flow of all nipples tested

and Harmer (2010) recommend the use of an artificial nipple that has a gradual transition from the tip to the base in order to cause the mouth to open wider. The infant will need to encompass a portion of the nipple base and should be able to maintain the mouth in a wide-open position with upper and lower lips flared out throughout the feeding. Clinicians will need to assure that the artificial nipple base is not too wide for the infant, causing overstretching of the mouth.

Because of these differences, which can sometimes be quite subtle, questions may arise about an infant's ability to correctly suckle at breast if he or she has been exposed to an artificial nipple that requires different sucking dynamics. This phenomenon has been referred to as nipple confusion or probably more accurately, nipple preference. Neifert, Lawrence, and Seacat (1995) defined nipple confusion as "an infant's difficulty in achieving the correct oral configuration, latching technique, and suckling pattern necessary for successful breastfeeding after bottle feeding or other exposure to an artificial nipple." The fact that nipple preference occurs is probably best illustrated by bottle-fed infants who have difficulty changing between bottle nipples of varying designs. Some of these infants will reject various brands of nipples until they find one that is acceptable to them. Although the term "confusion" may be inaccurate, it may be that it is the tactile and proprioceptive qualities of an object that influence or alter the infant's oral movements and acceptance (Wolf & Glass, 1992). These qualities may act as a "super-stimulus" and simply overwhelm an infant's sensitive mouth.

Some infants have no difficulty alternating between the breast and an artificial nipple. Others may experience difficulty in rapidly adapting to a change or may take time to learn a different behavior. A subset of infants may be unable to differentiate between the sucking movements required to extract milk relative to the differing types of nipples presented to them. According to Sakashita et al. (1996), "Bottle feeding is a non-physiological condition and the physiological behavior is replaced by an adaptive change, the sucking action." There is currently no way to predict which infants will have difficulty and which ones will transition between breast and bottle effortlessly. In an effort to prevent or reduce latch, suck, and numerous other problems attributed to artificial nipples, alternatives to bottles may be recommended. These devices can be used temporarily to deliver nutrition, may be selected to assist with latch-on, or may be necessary for longer periods of time to deliver nutrients while an infant learns to feed at breast. Common devices include tube feeding setups, cups, spoons, droppers, syringes, and paladai.

Tube feeding devices include commercial versions, such as the Supplemental Nursing System and the Starter Supplemental Nursing System (Medela, Inc.), the Lact-Aid Nursing Trainer System (Lactaid International), and the SuppleMate Infant Care (Maternal Concepts), that can be used for supplementation at the breast or with finger feeding. A gavage feeder can be used or a five French feeding tube inserted into a bottle through the artificial nipple may be used as a non-commercial type of supplementer. Tube feeding supplementers can be assembled from butterfly tubing (with the needle cut off) and a syringe. The size of the syringe will depend on the amount of supplement required. If an infant can latch to the breast, a tube feeding device for supplementation at the breast is preferable to other supplemental devices, as it allows active feeding at the breast, proper programming and strengthening of the oral and facial structures, protection of the maternal milk supply, and supplementation during or after breastfeedings. If an infant has difficulty latching to the breast or staying latched to the breast and generates low levels of vacuum, the supplementer tubing can be run under a nipple shield. The softer silastic tubing from the Supplemental Nutrition System or Lact-Aid Nursing Trainer may be preferable to tubing from a gavage feeder or five French feeding tubing which may be too stiff to be placed under a nipple shield. Such stiff tubing may interfere with adherence of the shield to the breast. Most mothers will tape the tubing to the breast to hold it in place while the baby feeds. Sterile paper tape can be used, but falls off when wet. Some mothers use a non-latex bandaid to hold the tubing in place. Tube placement can be on top of the nipple, but care must be taken when latching not to tip up the tubing above the infant's upper lip. Placing the tubing to the side or underneath the nipple may keep the tubing from interfering with the latch. The tip of the tubing should extend a little past the tip of the nipple, as the nipple and areola elongate when drawn into the baby's mouth. The baby, however, should not be sucking on the tubing like a straw. Pursed lips, dimpled cheeks, and a shallow latch are indicators that the baby is not attached properly. Placing the tubing under the nipple and/or positioning the end of the tubing slightly back from the tip of the nipple may help prevent or remedy this situation.

The Hazelbaker FingerFeeder (Aidan & Eva) can be used with one hand to finger feed an infant. Similarly acting devices can be created from gavage tubing, from a length of butterfly tubing (with the needle removed) attached to a 20 cc or 30 cc syringe (Edgehouse & Radzyminski, 1990), or a 36-inch length of five French tubing threaded through an artificial nipple on a feeding bottle (Newman, 1990). Finger feeding with any of these tubing devices utilizes the tubing attached to a caregiver's finger in the infant's mouth (Bull & Barger, 1987). Finger feeding may be chosen when the mother cannot be available for a feeding, when the nipples are too sore or damaged for direct breastfeeding, when the infant cannot latch and/ or use a tube feeding device at the breast, or to allow the mother to rest after a feeding. Finger feeding (rather than a bottle) allows the caregiver to better pace a feeding, provides the feel of real skin rather than silicone or latex, helps establish proper oral conformation, and does not allow intake of milk from compression only. Like an artificial nipple, a finger in the infant's mouth is a rigid entity. However, an infant must exert vacuum using similar oral activities as sucking at the breast and cannot obtain milk by compression only as on most artificial nipples.

The Supplemental Nursing System (Medela, Inc.) holds more milk than the other supplementation tools. It has three different sizes of tubing, small, medium, and large. It allows two lengths of tubing to be attached one to each breast and has a number of options to vary the milk flow rate. The tubes are attached to the valve in the cap of the semi-rigid plastic milk container. Raising or lowering the container by adjusting the neck cord allows a faster or slower flow, as does using the largest or smallest set of tubing. Generally, the medium-sized tubing is started running on one breast by unclamping that tube from a notch in the container cap.

The other breast's tubing is kept occluded in the cap's notch until ready to be used. Twins can be supplemented simultaneously when one length of tubing is taped to each breast. A faster flow can be obtained by unlatching the second tube and taping it pointing up, so that milk does not drain out of it. Both sets of tubing can be used on one breast for a faster flow and increased supplement volume, especially for an infant who cannot generate much or any vacuum. An infant who has low weight gain or has lost weight should be supplemented (ideally with expressed breastmilk) with as much as he will take at first. Once milk is left in the container, smaller amounts can be offered by reducing the supplement by half an ounce at each feeding every other day. As the infant's sucking efficiency improves, the supplementer can be hooked up, but run after a feeding, then run after every other feeding. Mothers may have mixed feelings about using this device or any of the supplementation devices. They can add time to the length of the feedings and must be cleaned after each use.

The Lact-Aid Nursing Trainer is somewhat complicated to assemble and clean. Care must be taken if using powdered formula, as any lumps in the formula can clog the tubing. This tool will help increase the mother's milk supply. The supplemental milk is placed in a plastic bag that hangs around the mother's neck. The bag can be gently pressed to increase milk flow, but should not be squeezed such that it overwhelms the infant. The bag of milk generally is hung a couple of inches above the nipple. It is important to make sure that the infant is properly latched with the tubing in his mouth if the tubing is placed on the underside of the nipple.

Mothers and families using tube-feeding devices usually do so on a temporary basis. The mother typically uses them to establish the infant at breast and/or supplement the infant at breast. However, some mothers use tube-feeding devices for longer-term breastfeeding, such as for adoptive nursing, if the mother has had a breast reduction or other surgery on the breasts, if she is experiencing insufficient breastmilk, or if the infant is not capable of feeding directly at the breast without assistance because of oral anomalies like cleft palate, genetic or anatomical problems, or neurological compromise. For longer-term supplementation, it may be easier if the mother uses a device with a larger fluid capacity. The devices that consist of a length of tubing and a syringe or the finger-feeding devices hold only small amounts of milk, which is ideal for the early days following birth. When using tube-feeding devices, small boluses can be effective if needed to help the infant initiate and sustain sucking, as flow regulates suck. Establishing milk flow in the infant's mouth will usually result in the baby swallowing and engaging in further sucking attempts. Flow rate can be adjusted to either augment or reduce the flow. If the infant is looking distressed, sputtering, coughing, or choking, then the flow needs to be reduced such that a comfortable ratio of sucking to swallowing is seen and the infant inhibits breathing only when swallowing. Although some mothers may find these devices awkward or inconvenient, they have been shown to be an effective tool in addressing selected breastfeeding problems in term and preterm infants, and extending the duration of breastfeeding (Oddy & Glenn, 2003; Borucki, 2005; Guoth-Gumberger, 2006; Both & Frischknecht, 2008).

Cup feeding has been utilized for decades as an alternative feeding method and for supplementation of breastfed infants. It allows the infant to pace his feeding, minimizes the risk of aspiration, reduces energy expenditure while feeding, and removes the risk of desaturation during a feeding episode. It can be done by both clinicians and parents. It provides a safe artificial method of feeding preterm and low-birth-weight infants until they are developmentally mature enough to obtain milk through exclusive breastfeeding (Marinelli, Burke, & Dodd, 2001). Cup feeding migrated from a supplementation or feeding method of preterm infants to those full-term infants who require supplementation assistance. Commercial infant-feeding cups are available in hard and soft plastic in varying shapes and sizes from Medela, Inc., Ameda, Maternal Concepts, and Foley. Some clinicians use a 28 ml medicine cup or a small party-favor-size plastic cup with a rounded rim. Cup feeding facilitates the participation of the masseter and temporalis muscles, similar to the functioning of these muscles during breastfeeding (Gomes, Trezza, Murade, & Padovani, 2006). Cup feeding of supplements to breastfed infants has been shown to be safe, resulting in a lower incidence of desaturation episodes (especially in preterm infants) and helping to prolong breastfeeding, particularly if multiple supplements are required (Rocha, Martinez, & Jorge, 2002; Howard et al., 1999; Howard et al., 2003). Abouelfettoh, Dowling, Dabash, Elguindy, and Seoud (2008) showed that preterm infants who were supplemented by cup demonstrated more mature breastfeeding behaviors when compared to bottle-fed infants over six weeks and had a significantly higher proportion of breastfeedings one week after discharge. Yilmaz, Caylan, Karacan, Bodur, and Gokay (2014) conducted a study to determine the effect of bottle and cup feeding on exclusive breastfeeding rates at hospital discharge and at three and six months in late preterm infants. Exclusive breastfeeding rates were significantly higher in the cup-supplemented infants compared to those infants supplemented with a bottle. There was no difference found between length of hospital stay between the bottle-fed and cup-fed groups. Mean weight gain in the first week of the study and mean feeding time on day seven of the study did not differ between the bottle-fed and cup-fed groups. Cup feeding, however, can be slow with some infants and involve spillage, which must be accounted for when feeding fragile preterm infants. Systematic reviews of older studies have not found nipple confusion to be affected by cup feeding (Flint, New, & Davies, 2007; Collins, Makrides, Gillis, & McPhee, 2008). Cup feeding in one study had the potential to delay discharge from the hospital for some preterm infants, but compliance with the assigned feeding method was poor and made identification of a real treatment effect less powerful (Collins, Makrides, Gillis, & McPhee, 2008). Cup feeding appears to be a relatively easy method of supplementation, but it does not protect or increase a mother's milk supply unless the mother is also expressing her milk. Clinicians will need to remain vigilant regarding milk production. Cup feeding also does not teach an infant to feed at the breast, but at least it requires activation of similar muscles used when breastfeeding. The cup should not be used in a manner that pours the milk into the infant's mouth. This provides the potential for aspiration and overwhelms the infant's ability to swallow. The proper technique is to allow the milk to only touch the lower lip, causing the infant to lick or sip the milk. The Foley Cup Feeder is a soft flexible cup with a rim extension that has a groove or channel on the extension that directs the milk into the small lip, or if tilted enough, will create a small stream of milk. As the cup is tilted, a small amount of milk flows into the rim extension, which is then placed on the infant's lower lip. The SuckleCup Infant Feeder is a soft flexible feeding cup that allows the edges to be squeezed together to regulate the flow of milk to the rim.

Small plastic spoons can be used to collect hand-expressed colostrum and spoon-feed to a newborn who is unable to latch onto the breast (Hoover, 1998). Hand expressing colostrum directly into the spoon rather than the collection bottle of a breast pump facilitates the capture of as much of the small amounts of colostrum as possible. Using a breast pump to collect colostrum for supplementation can often result in colostrum sticking to the sides of the collection container, making it very difficult to secure an appropriate volume of colostrum. When colostrum is collected into a spoon, it eliminates having to transfer the colostrum into another container or supplementer device, furthering the potential to preserve the volume of usable colostrum. The Medela Soft Feeder has a spoon-shaped spout at the end of a milk reservoir. Pre-wrapped disposable plastic spoons can be used as well as maroon spoons. Regular clean kitchen spoons can be used at home if the infant still requires small amounts of supplements following discharge. Maroon spoons are used by feeding therapists, come in two sizes, and have a narrow shallow bowl which is well suited for spoon-feeding a small infant. The volume of fluid that can be held in a regular teaspoon is 5 ml. Kumar, Dabas, and Singh (2010) studied spoon-feeding as a supplementing method and evaluated low-birth-weight infants' growth and transition to breastfeeding. They found that spoon-feeding was a feasible way to supplement these infants until they were fully established at breast.

Glass or plastic medicine droppers or soft plastic clinical droppers are useful to provide milk incentives at the breast for teaching latch-on (Figure 5.1).

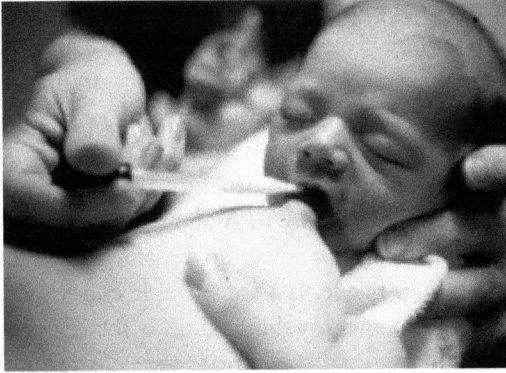

Figure 5.1. Dropper assist with latch on
Source: Courtesy of Marsha Walker, RN, IBCLC

Droppers can be used to provide small boluses of milk at the breast or for supplementing small amounts of milk when finger feeding. TB (tuberculin) syringes can be used for this purpose, or periodontal syringes may be selected to deliver larger quantities of milk on a temporary basis. A curved tip or periodontal syringe allows for a very precise control of milk flow. A paladai resembles a small gravy boat with a spout that is similar to cup feeding, but reduces the spillage common with cup feeding (Malhotra, Vishwambaran, Sundaram, & Narayanan, 1999). Use of a paladai in one study produced more spillage than the use of a bottle and increased feeding time in preterm infants (Aloysius & Hickson, 2007).

All alternative feeding methods have strengths and weaknesses (Table 5.4). Therefore, they must be selected with the goals of establishing or returning the infant to feedings at the breast while preserving the milk supply.

Table 5.4. Strengths and Limitations of Selected Alternative Feeding Devices

Tube Feeding Devices

Strengths

- All feeding opportunities are at the breast
- Shapes desired feeding behavior with consistent practice and positive reinforcement
- Reduces risk of faulty imprinting on an artificial nipple
- Can improve infant weight gain rapidly
- Facilitates milk production with frequent breast stimulation
- Provides milk flow into the infant's mouth which regulates sucking
- Can reduce feeding times and frustration

Limitations

- May be awkward, cumbersome, and unappealing
- May reinforce maternal feelings of inadequacy
- Requires close professional follow-up and monitoring
- Tube placement may interfere with latch or cause infant to suck on the tube like a straw
- Cleaning of parts may be time consuming
- Parts can break or be expensive for some parents

Finger Feeding

Strengths

- Helps provide proper mouth conformation for feeding at breast
- Requires the infant to open his mouth wide
- Keeps the tongue down, forward, and cupped
- Infant receives milk when sufficient vacuum is applied
- Prevents the infant from biting or compressing to obtain milk as from an artificial nipple
- Aids in suck training
- Proves a quick method for supplementing and can be done by anyone

Limitations

- A firm finger does not change shape with sucking
- An infant could become reliant on the firm nature of the finger
- If the finger is inserted into the infant's mouth through closed lips, he may not learn to draw the nipple and areola into his mouth

- There is no breast stimulation with finger feeding
- Mother will need to express milk

Syringe/Dropper Feeding

Strengths

- Can be used as an incentive to assist with latching to the breast
- Can help reinforce proper sucking
- Useful to create milk flow in the infant's mouth to establish and regulate sucking
- Helpful to use to reward sucking attempts and shape desired sucking behavior
- Avoids nipple preference from the use of an artificial nipple
- Can be used to supplement small amounts of milk

Limitations

- May need a second person to help if supplementation is being done at the breast
- Represents a foreign and firm object in the infant's mouth
- Potential for too forceful milk injection into the mouth, causing baby to choke
- Is a slow way to provide larger amounts of supplement

Bottle-feeding

Strengths

- A fast and easy way for an infant to obtain milk
- A more rapid method of providing larger amounts of supplement
- Does not require a large amount of time expenditure
- Anyone can feed the infant
- May need to be considered if long-term supplementation is necessary

Limitations

- May reduce the mother's desire to continue feeding at breast
- Requires mother to express milk
- Artificial nipple may weaken baby's suck, suppress the central grooving of the tongue, decrease masseter muscle activity and development
- May reinforce improper oral conformation making it difficult to return to the breast

- May induce bradycardia, apnea, and oxygen desaturation in some more vulnerable infants
- Can contribute to oral cavity alterations and malocclusions

Cup Feeding

Strengths

- Rapid method to supplement an infant that does not contribute to nipple preference as with an artificial nipple
- Allows the infant to pace his own feeding (Lang, 1994)
- Can decrease the amount of time gavage feeding is used
- May reduce oral defensiveness
- Requires tongue to move down and forward
- Does not result in breathing challenges or alterations or oxygen desaturation
- Can be used with term and preterm infants
- Anyone can supplement the infant
- Provides positive feeding experiences

Limitations

- Does not teach sucking at the breast
- Does not increase milk production and requires mother to express milk
- Infant may become so accustomed to cup feeding that he will not return to breast
- Caregivers may become so accustomed to cup feeding that breastfeeding is not encouraged
- Spillage can be significant and can cause difficulty if quantifying intake is necessary as with preterm or fragile infants
- Pouring milk into the infant's mouth can contribute to aspiration and loss of feeding skills

Supplementation should not be undertaken in a random or unplanned manner and should be conducted with specific therapeutic goals in mind. Documentation when supplementing should include the indication, route of delivery, type of supplement, and amount ingested by the infant. When a mother requests that her infant be supplemented, the clinician will need to ask why the mother is requesting this action, dispel any misconceptions, advise of potential risks and consequences, and educate other family members if they are the cause of the request. Mothers or staff may feel the need to supplement infants in the evening or at night, because many infants are unsettled at these times. Mothers may state they are "feeding all the time," that the infant does not appear to be getting enough, and that the infant does not fall asleep after feeding. Rather than giving the infant a bottle of formula, clinicians should first directly assess a feeding at breast, recommend techniques to improve milk transfer, and recognize that they may be observing a normal diurnal feeding pattern that is common during the hospital stay and beyond. Benson (2001) demonstrated that the frequency of feeding in infants during the first 60 hours after birth was lowest between 3:00 a.m. and 9:00 a.m., and then gradually increased throughout the day to the highest frequency between 9:00 p.m. and 3:00 a.m. This is the precise time that maternity unit staffing levels are at their lowest, lactation consultants may be unavailable, and family members have either gone home or are as tired as the mother. Evening and night staffing that includes lactation consultants, staff nurses with additional breastfeeding management expertise, and staffing ratios that allow for more time per patient might alleviate unnecessary supplementation and its resulting side effects. Judicious supplementation of human milk when medically indicated points the way to best practices and sustained breastfeeding.

Resources

Books and Pamphlets

Guoth-Gumberger, M. (2006). *Breastfeeding with the supplementary nursing system (SNS)*. Available at http://www.breastfeeding-support.de/eng/pub.htm

Genna, C.W. (2009). *Selecting and using breastfeeding tools*. Amarillo, TX, Hale Publishing.

Peterson, A., Harmer, M. (2010). *Balancing breast & bottle: reaching your breastfeeding goals*. Amarillo, TX: Hale Publishing.

Scripts for Clinicians

Hospital Breastfeeding Toolkit-Illinois

http://www.scribd.com/doc/118247333/Hospital-Breastfeeding-Toolkit-Illinois

University of Rochester Medical Center

http://www.urmc.rochester.edu/flrpp/breast-feeding-hospital-policy/toolkits/documents/FloorTools.pdf

Stanford Newborn Nursery

http://newborns.stanford.edu/Breastfeeding/PMGs.html

Supplementation Policies

California Department of Public Health

http://www.cdph.ca.gov/HealthInfo/healthyliving/childfamily/Pages/BFP-MdlHospToolkitPolicy8.aspx

Includes links to formula supplementing consent forms

Academy of Breastfeeding Medicine

http://www.bfmed.org/Media/Files/Protocols/Protocol%203%20English%20Supplementation.pdf

Antenatal Colostrum Expression

Cairns Health Service District 2008, *Protocol — Antenatal expression of colostrum for mothers with diabetes and other mothers whose babies are likely to have feeding difficulties*

http://home.ca.inter.net/~jfisher/docs/Appendix%201%20-%20Antenatal%20Expression.pdf

Stanford University Newborn Nursery video of hand expression
http://newborns.stanford.edu/Breastfeeding/HandExpression.html
Brochure: Breastfeeding—antenatal expression of colostrum
http://brochures.mater.org.au/Home/Brochures/Mater-Mothers-Hospital/Breastfeeding-antenatal-expression-of-colostrum

Alternative Devices for Supplementing the Breastfed Infant

Cups

Foley cup
Foley Development, Inc.
PO Box 50
Conway, MI 49722
888-463-2688
www.foleycup.com

Suckle cup
Maternal Concepts
130 North Public St.
Elmwood, WI 54740
800-310-5817
www.maternalconcepts.com

Ameda baby cup
Ameda
485 Half Day Rd., Suite 320
Buffalo Grove, IL 60089
877-992-6332
www.ameda.com

Soft Feeder
Medela, Inc.
1101 Corporate Dr.
McHenry, IL 60050
800-435-8316
www.medela.com

Flexi-Cut cup (uses a cutout design to prevent neck extension)
New Visions
1124 Roberts Mountain Rd.
Faber, VA 22938
800-606-7112
www.new-vis.com

Tube-feeding devices

Hazelbaker FingerFeeder
Aidan and Eva
5115 Olentangy River Rd
Columbus, OH 43235
614 451-1154
www.fingerfeeder.com/index.html
www.aidanandevapress.com

Lact-Aid International, Inc. (Lact-Aid nursing training device)
PO Box 1066
Athens, TN 37371
866 866-1239
www.lact-aid.com

Supplemental Nursing System
Medela, Inc.
1101 Corporate Dr.
McHenry, IL 60050
800-435-8316 or 1-815-363-1166
www.medela.com

SuppleMate Infant Care

Maternal Concepts

130 North Public St.

Elmwood, WI 54740

800-310-5817

www.maternalconcepts.com

Maroon spoons

New Visions

1124 Roberts Mountain Rd.

Faber, VA 22938

800-606-7112

www.new-vis.com

References

Aaltonen, J., Ojala, T., Laitinen, K., Poussa, T., Ozanne, S., & Isolauri, E. (2011). Impact of maternal diet during pregnancy and breastfeeding on infant metabolic programming: A prospective randomized controlled study. *European Journal of Clinical Nutrition, 65*, 10-19.

Abouelfettoh, A.M., Dowling, D.A., Dabash, S.A., Elguindy, S.R., & Seoud, I.A. (2008). Cup versus bottle feeding for hospitalized late preterm infants in Egypt: A quasi-experimental study. *International Breastfeeding Journal, 3*, 27.

Abrahams, S.W., & Labbok, M.H. (2009). Exploring the impact of the Baby-Friendly Hospital Initiative on trends in exclusive breastfeeding. *International Breastfeeding Journal, 29*,4:11.

Academy of Breastfeeding Medicine. (2009). Hospital guidelines for the use of supplementary feedings in the healthy term breastfed neonate. Clinical Protocol #3. Revised 2009. *Breastfeeding Medicine. 4*,175-182.

Adamkin, D.H., Committee on Fetus and Newborn, American Academy of Pediatrics. (2011). Clinical report-postnatal glucose homeostasis in late-preterm and term infants. *Pediatrics, 127*, 575-579.

Adlerberth, I., & Wold, A.E. (2009). Establishment of the gut microbiota in Western infants. *Acta Paediatrica, 98*, 229-238.

Aizawa, M., Mizuno, K., & Tamura, M. (2010). Neonatal sucking behavior- comparison of perioral movement during breastfeeding and bottle feeding. *Pediatric International, 52*, 104-108.

Akaba, K., Kimura,T., Sasaki, A., Tanabe, S, Ikegami, T., Hasimoto, M., et al. (1998). Neonatal hyperbilirubinemia and mutation of the bilirubin uridine diphosphate-glucuronosyltransferase gene: a common missense mutation among Japanese, Koreans, and Chinese. *Biochemistry & Molecular Biology International, 46*, 21-26.

Aloysius, A., & Hickson, M. (2007). Evaluation of paladai cup feeding in breast-fed preterm infants compared with bottle feeding. *Early Human Development, 83*, 619–621.

Al-Sahab, B., Feldman, M., Macpherson, A., Ohlsson, A., & Tamim, H. (2010). Which method of breastfeeding supplementation is best? The beliefs and practices of paediatricians and nurses. *Paediatric Child Health, 15*, 427-431.

American Academy of Family Physicians, AAFP Breastfeeding Advisory Committee. (2008). Breastfeeding, family physicians supporting (Position paper). http://www.aafp.org/about/ policies/all/breastfeeding-support.html

American Academy of Pediatrics, Section on Breastfeeding. (2012). Breastfeeding and the use of human milk. *Pediatrics, 129*, e827-e841.

American College of Nurse Midwives. (2011). Breastfeeding. http://midwife.org/ACNM/files/ ACNMLibraryData/UPLOADFILENAME/000000000248/Breastfeeding%20statement%20 May%202011.pdf

American College (Congress) of Obstetricians and Gynecologists. (2007). Breastfeeding: maternal and infant aspects. ACOG Committee Opinion No. 361. *Obstetrics and Gynecology, 109*, 479-480.

American Dietetic Association (Academy of Nutrition and Dietetics), James, D.C., & Lessen, R. (2009). Position of the American Dietetic Association: Promoting and supporting breastfeeding. Journal of the American Dietetic Association, 109, 1926-1942.

American Public Health Association. (2007). A call to action on breastfeeding: A fundamental public health issue. http://www.apha.org/advocacy/policy/policysearch/default.htm?id=1360

Apple, R.D. (1987). *Mothers and medicine: A social history of infant feeding 1890-1950.* Madison, WI: University of Wisconsin Press.

Backhed, F., Ding, H., Wang, T., Hooper, L.V., Koh, G.Y., Nagy, A., … Gordon, J.L. (2004). The gut microbiota as an environmental factor that regulates fat storage. *Proceedings of the National Academy of Science USA. 101*, 15718–15723.

Benson, S. (2001). What is normal? A study of normal breastfeeding dyads during the first sixty hours of life. *Breastfeeding Review, 9,* 27–32.

Bentley, M.E., Dee, D.L., & Jensen, J.L. (2003). Breastfeeding among low income, African American women: power, beliefs and decision making. *Journal of Nutrition, 133,* 305S-309S.

Bergman, N.J. (2013). Neonatal stomach volume and physiology suggest feeding at 1-h intervals. *Acta Paediatrica, 102,* 773-777.

Bertini, G., Dani, C., Tronchin, M., & Rubaltelli, F.F. (2001). Is breastfeeding really favoring early neonatal jaundice? *Pediatrics, 107,* e41-e45.

Bhutani, V.K., & Johnson, L. (2009). A proposal to prevent severe neonatal hyperbilirubinemia and kernicterus. *Journal of Perinatology, 29,* S61–S67.

Biro, M.A., Sutherland, G.A., Yelland, J.S., Hardy, P., & Brown, S.J. (2011). In-hospital formula supplementation of breastfed babies: A population-based survey. *Birth, 38,*302-310.

Black, L.S. (2001). Incorporating breastfeeding care into daily newborn rounds and pediatric office practice. *Pediatric Clinics of North America, 48,* 299–319.

Blomquist, H.K., Jonsbo, F., Serenius, F., & Persson, L.A. (1994). Supplementary feeding in the maternity ward shortens the duration of breastfeeding. *Acta Paediatrica Scandinavia, 83,* 1122–1126.

Bolton, T.A., Chow, T., Benton, P.A., & Olson, B.H. (2009). Characteristics associated with longer breastfeeding duration: An analysis of a peer counseling support program. *Journal of Human Lactation, 25,* 18-27.

Bonuck, K., Stuebe, A., Barnett, J., Labbok, M.H., Fletcher, J., & Bernstein, P.S. (2014). Effect of primary care intervention on breastfeeding duration and intensity. *American Journal of Public Health, 104* Suppl 1, S119-127.

Borucki, L.C. (2005). Breastfeeding mothers' experience using a supplemental feeding tube device: Finding an alternative. *Journal of Human Lactation, 21,* 429–438.

Both, D., & Frischknecht, K. (2008). *Breastfeeding: An illustrated guide to diagnosis and treatment.* Marrickville, NSW, Australia: Elsevier Australia.

Brisbane, J.M., & Giglia, R.C. (2013). Experiences of expressing and storing colostrum antenatally: A qualitative study of mothers in regional Western Australia. *Journal of Child Health Care,* DOI: 10.1177/1367493513503586 [Ahead of print].

Brodows, R.G., Pi-Sunyer, F.X., & Campbell, R.G. (1975). Sympathetic control of hepatic glycogenolysis during glucopenia in man. *Metabolism Clinical and Experimental, 24,* 617-624.

Brown, E.W., & Bosworth, A.W. (1922). Studies of infant feeding XVI. A bacteriological study of the feces and the food of normal babies receiving breastmilk. *American Journal of Diseases of Children, 23,* 243-258.

Bull, P., & Barger, J. (1987). Fingerfeeding with the SNS. *Rental Roundup,* 25–34.

Bullen, C.L., Tearle, P.V., & Stewart, M.G. (1977). The effect of humanized milks and supplemented breast feeding on the faecal flora of infants. *Journal of Medical Microbiology, 10,* 403–413.

Burdette, A.M. (2013). Neighborhood context and breastfeeding behaviors among urban mothers. *Journal of Human Lactation, 29,* 597-604.

Cabrera-Rubio, R., Collado, M.C., Laitinen, K., Salminen, S., Isolauri, E., & Mira, A. (2012). The human milk microbiome changes over lactation and is shaped by maternal weight and mode of delivery. *American Journal of Clinical Nutrition, 96,* 544-551.

Cadwell, K. (1997). Using the quality improvement process to affect breastfeeding protocols in United States hospitals. *Journal of Human Lactation, 13,* 5-9.

Cadwell, K., & Turner-Maffei, C. (2009). *Continuity of care in breastfeeding.* Sudbury, MA: Jones and Bartlett.

Caglar, M.K., Ozer, I., & Altugan F.S. (2006). Risk factors for excess weight loss and hypernatremia in exclusively breastfed infants. *Brazilian Journal of Medical Biology Research, 39,* 539–544.

Cantani, A., & Micera, M. (2005). Neonatal cow milk sensitization in 143 case-reports: Role of early exposure to cow's milk formula. *European Review for Medical and Pharmacological Sciences, 9,* 227–230.

Carvalho, J.C., & Mathias, R.S. (1994). Intravenous hydration in obstetrics. *International Anesthesiology Clinics, 32,* 103-115.

Castrucci, B.C., Hoover, K.L., Lim, S., & Maus, K.C. (2006). A comparison of breastfeeding rates in an urban birth cohort among women delivering infants at hospitals that employ and do not employ lactation consultants. *Journal of Public Health Management and Practice, 12,* 578-585.

Catassi, C., Bonucci, A., Coppa, G.V., Carlucci, A., & Giorgi, P.L. (1995). Intestinal permeability changes during the first month: Effect of natural versus artificial feeding. *Journal of Pediatric Gastroenterology and Nutrition, 21,* 383–386.

Centers for Disease Control and Prevention [CDC]. (2008). Breastfeeding-related maternity practices at hospitals and birth centers—United States, 2007. *Morbidity and Mortality Weekly Report, 57,* 621–625.

Centers for Disease Control and Prevention. (2013b). *mPINC results tables.* Accessed from http://www.cdc.gov/breastfeeding/data/mpinc/results-tables.htm

Centers for Disease Control and Prevention. (2013a) *Strategies to prevent obesity and other chronic diseases: The CDC guide to strategies to support breastfeeding mothers and babies.* Atlanta: U.S. Department of Health and Human Services.

Chang, R.J., Chou, H.C., Chang, Y.H., Chen, M.H., Chen, C.Y., Hsieh, W.S., & Tsao, P.N. (2012). Weight loss percentage prediction of subsequent neonatal hyperbilirubinemia in exclusively breastfed neonates. *Pediatrics & Neonatology, 53,* 41-44.

Chapman, T., Pincombe, J., & Harris, M. (2013). Antenatal breast expression: A critical review of the literature. *Midwifery. 29*, 203-210.

Chantry, C.J., Nommsen-Rivers, L.A., Peerson, J.M., Cohen, R.J., & Dewey, K.G. (2011). Excess weight loss in first-born breastfed newborns relates to maternal intrapartum fluid balance. *Pediatrics, 127*,e171-e179.

Chertok, I.R., Raz, I., Shoham, I., Haddad, H., & Wiznitzer, A. (2009). Effects of early breastfeeding on neonatal glucose levels of term infants born to women with gestational diabetes. *Journal of Human Nutrition and Dietetics, 22,* 166–169.

Chezem, J.C., Friesen, C., & Boettcher, J. (2003). Breastfeeding knowledge, breastfeeding confidence, and infant feeding plans: Effects on actual feeding practices. *Journal of Obstetric, Gynecologic, and Neonatal Nursing, 32,* 40–47.

Chezem, J.C., Friesen, C., Montgomery, P., Fortman, T., & Clark, H. (1998). Lactation duration: Influences of human milk replacements and formula samples on women planning postpartum employment. *Journal of Obstetric, Gynecologic, and Neonatal Nursing, 27,* 646-651.

Chou, H.C., Chen, M.H., Yang, H.I., Su, Y.N., Hsieh, W.S., Chen, C.Y., ... Tsao, P.N. (2011). 211G to a variation of UDP-glucuronosyl transferase 1A1 gene and neonatal breastfeeding jaundice. *Pediatric Research, 69,* 170-174.

Christensson, K., Siles, C., Moreno, L., Belaustequi, A., De La Fuente, P., Lagercrantz, H., ... Winberg, J. (1992). Temperature, metabolic adaption and crying in healthy full-term newborns cared for skin-to-skin or in a cot. *Acta Paediatrica, 81,* 488–493.

Christidis, I., Zotter, H., Rosegger, H., Engele, H., Kurz, R., & Kerbel, R. (2003). Infrared thermography in newborns: The first hour after birth. *Bynakol Geburtshilfliche Rundsch, 43,* 31–35.

Claud, E.C., & Walker, W.A. (2001). Hypothesis: Inappropriate colonization of the premature intestine can cause neonatal necrotizing enterocolitis. *FASEB Journal, 15,* 1398–1403.

Collado, M.C., Isolakuri, E., Laitinen, K., & Salminen, S. (2010). Effect of mother's weight on infant's microbiota acquisition, composition, and activity during early infancy: A prospective follow-up study initiated in early pregnancy. *American Journal of Clinical Nutrition, 92,* 1023-1030.

Collins, C.T., Makrides, M., Gillis, J., & McPhee, A. J. (2008). Avoidance of bottles during the establishment of breast feeds in preterm infants. *Cochrane Database Systematic Review, 8*(4), CD005252.

Cornblath, M., Hawdon, J.M., Williams, A.F., Aynsley-Green, A., Ward-Platt, M.P., Schwartz, R., & Kalhan, S.C. (2000). Controversies regarding definition of neonatal hypoglycemia: Suggested operational thresholds. *Pediatrics. 105,* 1141–1145.

Cornblath, M., Schwartz, R., Aynsley-Green, A., & Lloyd, J.K. (1990). Hypoglycemia in infancy: The need for a rational definition. *Pediatrics, 85,* 834–837.

Corriveau, S.K., Drake, E.E., Kellams, A.L., & Rovnyak, V.G. (2013). Evaluation of an office protocol to increase exclusivity of breastfeeding. *Pediatrics, 131,* 942-950.

Cotterman, K.J. (2004). Reverse pressure softening: A simple tool to prepare areola for easier latching during engorgement. *Journal of Human Lactation, 20,* 227-237.

Cottrell, B.H., & Detman, L.A. (2013). Breastfeeding concerns and experiences of African American mothers. *MCN American Journal of Maternal Child Nursing, 38,* 297-304.

Cox, S.G. (2006). Expressing and storing colostrum antenatally for use in the newborn period. *Breastfeeding Review, 14*, 11–16.

Cox, S. (2010). An ethical dilemma: Should recommending antenatal expressing and storing of colostrum continue? *Breastfeeding Review, 18*, 5-7.

Crivelli-Kovach, A., & Chung, E.K. (2011). An evaluation of hospital breastfeeding policies in the Philadelphia metropolitan area 1994-2009: A comparison with the Baby Friendly Hospital Initiative 10 Steps. *Breastfeeding Medicine, 6*,77-84.

Crossland, D.S., Richmond, S., Hudson, M., Smith, K., & Abu-Harb, M. (2008). Weight change in the term baby in the first 2 weeks of life. *Acta Paediatrica, 97*,425-429.

Dabard, J., Bridonneau, C., Phillipe, C., Anglade, P., Molle, D., Nardi, M., … Fons, M. (2001). A new lantibiotic produced by a Ruminococcus gnavus strain isolated from human feces. *Applied Environmental Microbiology, 67*, 4111–4118.

Dahlenburg, G.W., Burnell, R.H., & Braybrook, R. (1980). The relation between cord serum sodium levels in newborn infants and maternal intravenous therapy during labor. *British Journal of Obstetrics and Gynaecology, 87*, 519–522.

Daly, S.E.J., Owens, R.A., & Hartmann, P.E. (1993). The short-term synthesis and infant-regulated removal of milk in lactating women. *Experimental Physiology, 78*, 209–220.

DaMota, K., Banuelos, J., Goldbronn, J., Vera-Beccera, L.E., & Heinig, M.J. (2012). Maternal request for in-hospital supplementation of healthy breastfed infants among low-income women. *Journal of Human Lactation, 28*, 476-482.

Davanzo, R., Cannioto, Z., Ronfani, L., Monasta, L., & Demarini, S. (2013). Breastfeeding and neonatal weight loss in healthy term infants. *Journal of Human Lactation, 29*, 45-53.

De Carvalho, M., Hall, M., & Harvey, D. (1981). Effects of water supplementation on physiological jaundice in breastfed babies. *Archives of Disease in Childhood, 56*, 568–569.

De Carvalho, M., Klaus, M. H., & Merkatz, R.B. (1982). Frequency of breastfeeding and serum bilirubin concentration. *American Journal of Disease in Childhood, 136*, 737–738.

De Carvalho, M., Robertson, S., & Klaus, M. (1985). Fecal bilirubin excretion and serum bilirubin concentrations in breastfed and bottle-fed infants. *Journal of Pediatrics, 107*, 786–790.

De Rooy, L., & Hawdon, J. (2002). Nutritional factors that affect the postnatal adaptation of full-term small- and large-for gestational-age infants. *Pediatrics, 109*, e42.

Declercq, E.R., Sakala, C., Corry, M.P., Applebaum, S., & Herrlich, A. (2013). *Listening to mothers III: Pregnancy and birth.* New York: Childbirth Connection.

De Moura, E.G., Lisboa, P.C., & Passos, M.C. (2008). Neonatal programming of neuroimmunomodulation—role of adipocytokines and neuropeptides. *Neuroimmunomodulation. 15*, 176–188.

Dennis, C.L. (1999). Theoretical underpinnings of breastfeeding confidence: A self-efficacy framework. *Journal of Human Lactation, 15*, 195-201.

Dewey, K.G., Nommsen-Rivers, L.A., Heinig, M.J., & Cohen, R.J. (2003). Risk factors for suboptimal infant breastfeeding behavior, delayed onset of lactation, and excess neonatal weight loss. *Pediatrics, 112*, 607-619.

Di Frisco, E., Goodman, K.E., Budin, W.C., Lilienthal, M.W., Kleinman, A., & Holmes, B. (2011). Factors associated with exclusive breastfeeding 2 to 4 weeks following discharge from a large, urban, academic medical center striving for Baby-Friendly designation. *Journal of Perinatal Education, 20*, 28-35.

Di Mauro, A., Neu, J., Riezzo, G., Raimondi, F., Martinelli, D., Francavilla, R., & Indrio, F. (2013). Gastrointestinal function development and microbiota. *Italian Journal of Pediatrics, 39*, 15. http://www.ijponline.net/content/39/1/15

Drewett, R.F., Woolridge, M.W., Jackson, D.A., Imong, S.M., Mangklabruks, A., Wongsawasdii, L., ... Baum, J.D. (1989). Relationships between nursing patterns, supplementary food intake and breast milkbreastmilk intake in a rural Thai population. *Early Human Development, 20*, 13–23.

Durand, R., Hodges, S., LaRock, S., Lund, L., Schmid, S., Swick, D., ... Perez, A. (1997). The effect of skin-to-skin breastfeeding in the immediate recovery period on newborn thermoregulation and blood glucose values. *Neonatal Intensive Care, March/April*, 23–29.

Edgehouse, L., & Radzyminski, S.G. (1990). A device for supplementing breastfeeding. *MCN, 15*, 34–35.

Eidelman, A.I. (2001). Hypoglycemia and the breastfed neonate. *Pediatric Clinics of North America, 48*, 377–387.

Ekstrom, A., Widstrom, A.M., & Nissen, E. (2003). Duration of breastfeeding in Swedish primiparous and multiparous women. *Journal of Human Lactation, 19*, 172–178.

Fadavi, S., Punwani, I.C., Jain, L., & Vidyasagar, D. (1997). Mechanics and energetics of nutritive sucking: A functional comparison of commercially available nipples. *Journal of Pediatrics, 130*, 740–745.

Fantuzzi, G. (2005). Adipose tissue, adipokines, and inflammation. *Journal of Allergy Clinical Immunology, 115*, 911, –919.

Favier, C.F., Vaughan, E.E., De Vos, W.M., & Akkermans, A.D.L. (2002). Molecular monitoring of succession of bacterial communities in human neonates. *Applied and Environmental Microbiology, 68*, 219-226.

Ferrante, A., Silvestri, R., & Montinaro, C. (2006). The importance of choosing the right feeding aids to maintain breastfeeding after interruption. *International Journal Orofacial Myology, 32*, 58–67.

Fildes, V.A. (1986). *Breasts, bottles and babies: A history of infant feeding.* Edinburgh: Edinburgh University Press.

Fitzpatrick, E., Dennison, B.A., Welge, S.B., Hisgen, S., Boyce, P.S., & Waniewski, P.A. (2013). Development of the breastfeeding quality improvement in hospitals learning collaborative in New York state. *Breastfeeding Medicine, 8*, 263-272.

Flaherman, V.J., Aby, J., Burgos, A.E., Lee, K.A., Cabana, M.D., & Newman, T.B. (2013). Effect of early limited formula on duration and exclusivity of breastfeeding in at-risk infants: An RCT. *Pediatrics, 131*, 1059-1065.

Flaherman, V.J., Bokser, S., & Newman, T.B. (2010). First-day newborn weight loss predicts in-hospital weight nadir for breastfeeding infants. *Breastfeeding Medicine, 5*, 165-168.

Flaherman, V.J., Kuzniewicz, M.W., Li, S., Walsh, E., McCulloch, C.E., & Newman, T.B. (2013). First-day weight loss predicts eventual weight nadir for breastfeeding newborns. *Archives of Disease in Childhood Fetal and Neonatal Edition, 98*, F488-F492.

Flint, A., New, K., & Davies, M.W. (2007). Cup feeding versus other forms of supplemental enteral feeding for newborn infants unable to fully breastfeed. *Cochrane Database Systematic Review,* (2):CD005092.

Forster, D.A., McEgan, K., Ford, R., Moorhead, A., Opie, G., Walker, S., & McNamara, C. (2011). Diabetes and antenatal milk expressing: A pilot project to inform the development of a randomised controlled trial. *Midwifery. 27,* 209-214.

Furman, L. (2013). Early limited formula is not ready for prime time. *Pediatrics, 131,* 1182-1183.

Gagnon, A.J., Leduc, G., Waghorn, K., Yang, H., & Platt, R.W. (2005). In-hospital formula supplementation of healthy breastfeeding newborns. *Journal of Human Lactation, 21,* 397–405.

Garrison, K.L., Byrne, J.A.C, & Moore, F. (2009). *Scripting: A guide for nurses.* Marblehead, MA: HCPro, Inc.

Gartner, L.M., & Herschel, M. (2001). Jaundice and breastfeeding. *Pediatric Clinics of North America, 48,* 389–399.

Geddes, D.T., Sakalidis, V.S., Hepworth, A.R., McClellan, H.L., Kent, J.C., Lai, C.T., & Hartmann, P.E. (2012). Tongue movement and intra-oral vacuum of term infants during breastfeeding and feeding from an experimental teat that released milk under vacuum only. *Early Human Development, 88,* 443-449.

Gerstley, J.R., Howell, K.M., & Nagel, B.R. (1932). Some factors influencing the fecal flora of infants. *American Journal of Diseases of Children, 43,* 555-565.

Glover, J, & Sandilands, M. (1990). Supplementation of breastfeeding infants and weight loss in hospital. *Journal of Human Lactation, 6,* 163-166.

Goldfield, E.C., Richardson, M.J., Lee, K.G., & Margetts, S. (2006). Coordination of sucking, swallowing, and breathing and oxygen saturation during early infant breastfeeding and bottle-feeding. *Pediatric Research, 60,* 450–455.

Goldstein, I., Reece, E.A., Yarkoni, S., Wan, M., Green, J.L., & Hobbins, J.C. (1987).Growth of the fetal stomach in normal pregnancies. *Obstetrics & Gynecology, 70,* 641-644.

Gomes, C.F., Trezza, E.M.C., Murade, E.C.M., & Padovani, C.R. (2006). Surface electromyography of facial muscles during natural and artificial feeding of infants. *Journal Pediatrics (Rio J), 82,* 103–109.

Gosalbes, M.J., Llop, S., Valles, Y., Moya, A., Ballester, F., & Francino, M.P. (2013). Meconium microbiota types dominated by lactic acid or enteric bacteria are differentially associated with maternal eczema and respiratory problems in infants. *Clinical & Experimental Allergy, 43,* 198-211.

Gourley, G.R., Li, Z., Kreamer, B.L., & Kosorok, M.R. (2005).A controlled, randomized, double-blind trial of prophylaxis against jaundice among breastfed newborns. *Pediatrics, 116,* 385-391.

Gronlund, M.M., Arvilommi, H., Kero, P., Lehtonen, O.P., & Isolauri, E. (2000). Importance of intestinal colonization in the maturation of humoral immunity in early infancy: A prospective follow up study of healthy infants 0-6 months. *Archives of Disease in Childhood Fetal and Neonatal Edition, 83,* F186-F192.

Grossman, X., Chaudhuri, J.H., Feldman-Winter, L., & Merewood, A. (2012). Neonatal weight loss at a US Baby-Friendly hospital. *Journal of the Academy of Nutrition and Dietetics, 112,* 410-413.

Guaraldi, F., & Salvatori, G. (2012). Effect of breast and formula feeding on gut microbiota shaping in newborns. *Frontiers in Cellular and Infection Microbiology, 2,* 94.

Guoth-Gumberger, M. (2006). *Breastfeeding with the supplementary nursing system (SNS)*. Available at http://www.breastfeeding-support.de/eng/pub.htm

Gurneesh, S., & Ellora, D. (2009). Effect of antenatal expression of breast milk at term to improve lactational performance: A prospective study. *Journal of Obstetrics Gynecology India, 59*, 308-311.

Halamek, L.P., & Stevenson, D.K. (1996). Neonatal jaundice and liver disease. In: Fanarof A., Martin, R., eds. *Neonatal-perinatal medicine: Diseases of the fetus and infant*. Vol. 2, 6th ed. St. Louis, MO: Mosby-Year Book; pp. 1345–1389.

Hall, R.T., Mercer, A.M., Teasley, S.L., McPherson, D.M., Simon, S.D., Santos, S.R., ... Hipsh, N.E. (2002). A breast-feeding assessment score to evaluate the risk for cessation of breast-feeding by 7 to 10 days of age. *Journal of Pediatrics,141*, 659-64.

Harris, D.L., Weston, P.J., & Harding, J.E. (2012). Incidence of neonatal hypoglycemia in babies identified as at risk. *Journal of Pediatrics, 161*, 787-791.

Hata, T., Tanaka, H., Noguchi, J., Inubashiri, E., Yanagihara, T., & Kondoh, S. (2010). Three-dimensional sonographic volume measurement of the fetal stomach. *Ultrasound in Medicine & Biology, 36*, 1808-1812.

Hawdon, J.M., Ward-Platt, M.P., & Aynsley-Green, A. (1992). Patterns of metabolic adaptation for term and preterm infants in the first neonatal week. *Archives of Disease in Childhood, 67*, 357–365.

Heinig, M.J., Banuelos, J., Goldbronn, J., & Kampp, J. (2009). *Fit WIC baby behavior study*. UC Davis Human Lactation Center, Davis, California. http://www.nal.usda.gov/wicworks/Sharing_Center/spg/CA_report2006.pdf

Herrera, A.J. (1984). Supplemented versus unsupplemented breastfeeding. *Perinatology/Neonatology, 8*, 70–71.

Higgins, J., Gleeson, R., Holohan, M., Cooney, C., & Darling, M. (1996). Maternal and neonatal hyponatremia: A comparison of Hartmann's solution with 5% dextrose for the delivery of oxytocin in labour. *European Journal of Obstetrics Gynaecology Reproductive Biology, 68*, 47–48.

Hill, P.D., Humenick, S.S., Brennan, M.L., & Woolley, D. (1997). Does early supplementation affect long-term breastfeeding? *Clinical Pediatrics (Phila), 36*, 345-350.

Hirth, R., Weitkamp, T., & Dwivedi, A. (2012). Maternal intravenous fluids and infant weight. *Clinical Lactation, 3*, 59-63.

Hoddinott. P., Craig, L.C., Britten, J., & McInnes, R.M. (2012). A serial qualitative interview study of infant feeding experiences: Idealism meets realism. *BMJ Open, 14*, 2 (2):e000504.

Holmes, A.V. (2013). Establishing successful breastfeeding in the newborn period. *Pediatric Clinics of North America, 60*, 147-168.

Holtrop, P.C., Madison, K.A., Kiechle, F.L., Karcher, R.E., & Batton, D.G. (1990). A comparison of chromogen test strip (Chemstrip bG) and serum glucose values in newborns. *American Journal of Disease in Childhood, 144*, 183–185.

Hoover, K. (1996). Visual assessment of the baby's wide open mouth. *Journal of Human Lactation, 12*, 9.

Hoover, K. (1998). Supplementation of the newborn by spoon in the first 24 hours. *Journal of Human Lactation, 14*, 245.

Hopkins, M.J., Macfarlane, G.T., Furrie, E., Fite, A., & Macfarlane, S. (2005). Characterisation of intestinal bacteria in infant stools using real-time PCR and northern hybridization analyses. *FEMS Microbiology Ecology, 54*, 77–85.

Hornell, A., Hofvander, Y., & Kylberg, E. (2001). Solids and formula: Association with pattern and duration of breastfeeding. *Pediatrics, 107*, e38.

Host, A. (1991). Importance of the first meal on the development of cow's milk allergy and intolerance. *Allergy Proceedings, 10*, 227–232.

Host, A., Husby, S., & Osterballe, O. (1988). A prospective study of cow's milk allergy in exclusively breastfed infants. *Acta Paediatrica Scandinavia, 77*, 663–670.

Howard, C.R., de Blieck, E.A., ten Hoopen, C.B., Howard, F.M., Lanphear, B.P., & Lawrence, R.A. (1999). Physiologic stability of newborns during cup- and bottle-feeding. *Pediatrics, 104*, 1204–1207.

Howard, C.R., Howard, F.M., Lanphear, B., Eberly, S., deBlieck, E.A., Oakes, D., & Lawrence, R.A. (2003). Randomized clinical trial of pacifier use and bottle-feeding or cupfeeding and their effect on breastfeeding. *Pediatrics, 111*, 511–518.

Huang, Y.Y., Gau, M.L., Huang, C.M., & Lee, J.T. (2009). Supplementation with cup-feeding as a substitute for bottle-feeding to promote breastfeeding. *Chang Gung Medical Journal, 32*, 423–431.

Inoue, I., Sakashita, R., & Kamegai, T. (1995). Reduction of masseter muscle activity in bottle-fed babies. *Early Human Development, 42*, 185–193.

Ishihara, T., Kaito, M., Takeuchi, K., Gabazza, E.C., Tanaka, Y., Higuchi, K., … Adachi, Y. (2001). Role of UGT1A1 mutation in fasting hyperbilirubinemia. *Journal of Gastroenterology Hepatology, 16*, 678-682.

Isolauri, E. (2012). Development of healthy gut microbiota early in life. *Journal of Paediatrics and Child Health, 48*, (Suppl. 3), 1-6.

Itoh, S., Kondo, M., Kusaka, T., Isobe, K., & Onishi, S. (2001). Differences in transcutaneous bilirubin readings in Japanese term infants according to feeding method. *Pediatrics International*, 43,12-15.

Iyer, N.P., Srinivasan, R., Evans, K., Ward, L., Cheung, W.Y., & Matthes, J.W. (2008). Impact of early weighing policy on neonatal hypernatraemic dehydration and breastfeeding. *Archives of Disease in Chilhood, 93*, 297–299.

Jacobs, L.A., Dickinson, J.E., Hart, P.D., Doherty, D.A., & Faulkner, S.J. (2007). Normal nipple position in term infants measured on breastfeeding ultrasound. *Journal of Human Lactation, 23*, 52–59.

Jimenez, E., Marin, M.L., Martin, R., Odriozola, J.M., Olivares, M., Xaus, J., … Rodriguez, J.M. (2008). Is meconium from healthy newborns actually sterile? *Research in Microbiology, 159*, 187-193.

Johnson, J.D. (1992). Jaundice in Navajo neonates. *Clinical Pediatrics (Phila), 31*, 716-718.

Jones, J.R., Kogan, M.D., Singh, G.K., Dee, D.L., & Grummer-Strawn, L.M. (2011). Factors associated with exclusive breastfeeding in the United States. *Pediatrics, 128*, 1117-1125.

Kair, L.R., Kenron, D., Etheredge, K., Jaffe, A.C., & Phillipi, C.A. (2013). Pacifier restriction and exclusive breastfeeding. *Pediatrics, 131*, e1101-e1107.

Kalliomaki, M., Collado, M.C., Salminen, S., Isolauri, E. (2008). Early differences in fecal microbiota composition in children may predict overweight. *American Journal of Clinical Nutrition, 87*, 534–538.

Kalliomaki, M., Kirjavainen, P., Eerola, E., Kero, P., Salminen, S., & Isolauri, E. (2001). Distinct patterns of neonatal gut microflora in infants developing or not developing atopy. *Journal of Allergy Clininical Immunology, 107*, 129–134.

Kaplan, M., & Eidelman, A.I. (1985). Improved prognosis in severely hypothermic newborns treated by rapid rewarming. *Journal of Pediatrics, 105*, 515–518.

Kaufman, L., Deenadayalan, S., & Karpati, A. (2010). Breastfeeding ambivalence among low-income African American and Puerto Rican women in North and Central Brooklyn. *Maternal Child Health Journal, 14*, 696-704.

Keppler, A.B. (1988). The use of intravenous fluids during labor. *Birth, 15*, 75–79.

Keren, R., Bhutani, V.K., Luan, X., Nihtianova, S., Cnaan, A., & Schwartz, J.S. (2005). Identifying newborns at risk of significant hyperbilirubinaemia: A comparison of two recommended approaches. *Archives of Disease in Childhood, 90*, 415-421.

Kernesiuk, N.L., Levchik, E.I., & Vilkova, I.V. (1997). Changes in the size of the stomach and its sections in human early postnatal ontogeny. *Morfologiia, 111*, 81-84.

Konetzny, G., Bucher, H.U., & Arlettaz, R. (2009). Prevention of hypernatraemic dehydration in breastfed newborn infants by daily weighing. *European Journal of Pediatrics, 168*, 815-818.

Kumar, A., Dabas, P., & Singh, B. (2010). Spoon feeding results in early hospital discharge of low birth weight babies. *Journal of Perinatology, 30*, 209-217.

Kurinij, N., & Shiono, P.H. (1991). Early formula supplementation of breastfeeding. *Pediatrics. 88*, 745–750.

Kusuma, S., Agrawal, S.K., Kumar, P., Narang, A., & Prasad, R. (2009). Hydration status of exclusively and partially breastfed near-term newborns in the first week of life. *Journal of Human Lactation, 25*, 280-286.

Lambrecht, L., Robberecht, E., Deschynkel, K., & Afschrift, M. (1988). Ultrasonic evaluation of gastric clearing in young infants. *Pediatric Radiology, 18*, 314–318.

Lamp, J.M., & Macke, J.K. (2010). Relationships among intrapartum maternal fluid intake, birth type, neonatal output, and neonatal weight loss during the first 48 hours after birth. *Journal of Obstetric Gynecologic and Neonatal Nursing, 39*, 169-177.

Lang, S. (1994). Cup-feeding: An alternative method. *Midwives Chronicle Nursing Notes, 107*, 171–176.

Levenstein, H. (2003). *Revolution at the table: The transformation of the American diet.* Berkeley, CA: University of California Press.

Ley, R., Backhed, F., Turnbaugh, P., Lozupone, C., Knight, R., & Gordon, J. (2005). Obesity alters gut microbial ecology. *Proceedings of the National Academy of Science USA. 102*, 11070–11075.

Livingstone, V.H., Willis, C.E., Abdel-Wareth, L., Thiessen, P., & Lockitch, G. (2000). Neonatal hypernatremic dehydration associated with breastfeeding malnutrition: Retrospective survey. *Canadian Medical Association Journal, 162*, 647–652.

Loke, A.Y., & Chan, L.K.S. (2013). Maternal breastfeeding self-efficacy and the breastfeeding behaviors of newborns in the practice of exclusive breastfeeding. *Journal of Obstetric, Gynecologic & Neonatal Nursing, 42*, 672-684.

Lucas, A. (1998). Programming by early nutrition: An experimental approach. *Journal of Nutrition, 128(2 Suppl)*, 401S–406S.

Macdonald, P.D., Ross, S.R., Grant, L., & Young, D. (2003). Neonatal weight loss in breast and formula fed infants. *Archives of Disease Childhood Fetal and Neonatal Edition, 88*, F472–F476.

Mackie, R.I., Sghir, A., & Gaskins, H.R. (1999). Developmental microbial ecology of the neonatal gastrointestinal tract. *American Journal of Clinical Nutrition, 69*, 1035S-1045S.

Maheshwari, A. & Zemlin, M. (2009). Ontogeny of the intestinal immune system. *Haematologica Reports, 2*, 10, 18-26.

Malhotra, N., Vishwambaran, L., Sundaram, K.R., & Narayanan, I. (1999). A controlled trial of alternative methods of oral feeding in neonates. *Early Human Development, 54*, 29–38.

Manganaro, R., Mami, C., Marrone, T., Marseglia, L., & Gemelli, M. (2001). Incidence of dehydration and hypernatremia in exclusively breastfed infants. *Pediatrics, 139*,673-675.

Marinelli, K.A., Burke, G.S., & Dodd, V.L. (2001). A comparison of the safety of cupfeedings and bottlefeedings in premature infants whose mothers intend to breastfeed. *Journal of Pediatrics, 21*, 350-355.

Martens, P.J., & Romphf, L. (2007). Factors associated with newborn in-hospital weight loss: Comparisons by feeding method, demographics, and birthing procedures. *Journal of Human Lactation, 23*, 233–241.

Mathew, O.P. (1988). Nipple units for newborn infants: A functional comparison. *Pediatrics, 81*, 688–691.

Mathew, O.P. (1990). Determinants of milk flow through nipple units: Role of hole size and nipple thickness. *American Journal of Diseases of Children, 144*, 222–224.

Merewood, A., Mehta, S.D., Chamberlain, L.B., Philipp, B.L., & Bauchner, H. (2005). Breast feeding rates in US Baby-Friendly hospitals: Results of a national survey. *Pediatrics, 116*, 628-34.

Merry, H., & Montgomery, A. (2000). Do breastfed babies whose mothers have had labor epidurals lose more weight in the first 24 hours of life? *Academy of Breastfeeding Medicine News and Views, 6*, 21.

Mikiel-Kostyra, K., & Mazur, J. (1999). Hospital policies and their influence on newborn body weight. *Acta Paediatrica, 88*, 72-75.

Mizuno, K., & Ueda, A. (2006). Changes in sucking performance from nonnutritive sucking to nutritive sucking during breast and bottle-feeding. *Pediatric Research, 59*, 728–731.

Morelli, L. (2008). Postnatal development of intestinal microflora as influenced by infant nutrition. *Journal of Nutrition, 138*, 1791S–1795S.

Moritz, M.L., Manole, M., Bogen, D.L., & Ayus, J.C. (2005). Breastfeeding-associated hypernatremia: Are we missing the diagnosis? *Pediatrics, 116*, e343–e347.

Morton, J.A. (1994). The clinical usefulness of breast milk sodium in the assessment of lactogenesis. *Pediatrics, 93*, 802-806.

Moscone, S.R., & Moore, M.J. (1993). Breastfeeding during pregnancy. *Journal of Human Lactation, 9*, 83-88.

Mountzouris, K.C., McCartney, A.L., & Gibson, G.R. (2002). Intestinal microflora of human infants and current trends for its nutritional modulation. *British Journal of Nutrition, 87*, 405-420.

Mulder, P.J., Johnson, T.S., & Baker, L.C. (2010). Excessive weight loss in breastfed infants during the postpartum hospitalization. *Journal of Obstetric Gynecologic and Neonatal Nursing, 39*, 15-26.

Nagata, S., Koyanagi, T., Fukushima, S., Akazawa, K., & Nakano, H. (1994). Change in the three-dimensional shape of the stomach in the developing human fetus. *Early Human Development, 37*, 27–38.

Naveed, M., Manjunath, C., & Sreenivas, V. (1992). An autopsy study of relationship between perinatal stomach capacity and birth weight. *Indian Journal of Gastroenterology, 11*, 156–158.

Neifert, M.R. (1998). The optimization of breastfeeding in the perinatal period. *Clinics in Perinatology, 25*, 303–326.

Neifert, M.R. (1999). Clinical aspects of lactation: Promoting breastfeeding success. *Clinics in Perinatology, 26*, 281–306.

Neifert, M.R. (2001). Prevention of breastfeeding tragedies. *Pediatric Clinics of North America, 48*, 273–297.

Neifert, M.R., Lawrence R., & Seacat, J. (1995). Nipple confusion: Toward a formal definition. *Journal of Pediatrics, 126*, S125–S129.

Neu, J., & Walker, W.A. (2011). Necrotizing enterocolitis. *New England Journal of Medicine, 364*, 255-264.

Newburg, D.S., & Walker, W.A. (2007). Protection of the neonate by the innate immune system of developing gut and of human milk. *Pediatric Research, 61*, 2–8.

Newman, J. (1990). Breastfeeding problems associated with the early introduction of bottles and pacifiers. *Journal of Human Lactation, 6*, 59–63.

Newton, K.N., Chaudhuri, J., Grossman, X., & Merewood, A. (2009). Factors associated with exclusive breastfeeding among Latina women giving birth at an inner-city Baby Friendly hospital. *Journal of Human Lactation, 25*, 28-33.

Nicoll, A., Ginsburg, R., & Tripp, J.H. (1982). Supplementary feeding and jaundice in newborns. *Acta Paediatrica Scandinavia, 71*, 759–761.

Nichols, J., Schutte, N.S., Brown, R.F., Dennis, C.S., & Price, I. (2009). The impact of a self-efficacy intervention on short-term breastfeeding outcomes. *Health Education & Behavior, 36*, 250-258.

Noel-Weiss, J., Courant, G., & Woodend, A.K. (2008). Physiological weight loss in the breastfed neonate: A systematic review. *Open Medicine, 2*, 11–22.

Noel-Weiss, J., Woodend, A.K., Peterson, W.E., Gibb, W., & Groll, D.L. (2011). An observational study of associations among maternal fluids during parturition, neonatal output, and breastfed newborn weight loss. *International Breastfeeding Journal, 6*, 9.

Nowak, A.J., Smith, W.L., & Erenberg, A. (1994). Imaging evaluation of artificial nipples during bottle feeding. *Archives Pediatric Adolescent Medicine, 148*, 40–42.

Oddie, S.J., Craven, V., Deakin, K., Westman, J., & Scally, A. (2013). Severe neonatal hypernatremia: A population based study. *Archives Disease Children Fetal Neonatal Edition, 98*, F384-387.

Oddy, W.H., & Glenn, K. (2003). Implementing the Baby Friendly Hospital Initiative: The role of finger feeding. *Breastfeeding Review, 11*, 5-10.

Okechukwu A.A, & Okolo, A.A. (2006). Exclusive breastfeeding frequency during the first seven days of life in term neonates. *Nigerian Postgraduate Medical Journal, 13*, 309-312.

Okumus, N., Atalay, Y., Onal, E.E., Turkyilmaz, C., Senel, S., Gunaydin, B., … Unal, S. (2011). The effects of delivery route and anesthesia type on early postnatal weight loss in newborns: The role of vasoactive hormones. *Journal of Pediatric Endocrinology Metabolism, 24*, 45-50.

Pados, B., Estrem, H., Nix, W.B., Park, J., & Thoyre, S. (2013). Milk flow rates from bottle nipples. Paper session A-1: Care of newborns and infants. Eastern Nursing Research Society, 25th Annual Scientific Session. April 17-19, Boston, Massachusetts.

Penn, A.H., Altshuler, A.E., Small, J.W., Taylor, S.F., Dobkins, K.R., & Schmid-Schonbein, G.W. (2012). Digested formula but not digested fresh human milk causes death of intestinal cells in vitro: Implications for necrotising enterocolitis. *Pediatric Research, 72*, 560-567.

Perrier, C., & Corthesy, B. (2011). Gut permeability and food allergies. *Clinical and Experimental Allergy, 41*, 20-28.

Perrine, C.G., Scanlon, K.S., Li, R., Odom, E., & Grummer-Strawn, L.M. (2012). Baby-Friendly hospital practices and meeting exclusive breastfeeding intention. *Pediatrics, 130*, 54-60.

Perrine, C.G., Shealy, K.R., Scanlon, K.S., Grummer-Strawn, L.M., & Galuska, D.A. (2011). Vital signs: Hospital practices to support breastfeeding – United States, 2007 and 2009. *Morbidity and Mortality Weekly Report, 60(30)*, 1020-1025.

Peterson, A. & Harmer, M. (2010). Balancing breast and bottle. Amarillo, TX: Hale Publishing.

Petrova, A., Hegyi, T., & Mehta, R. (2007). Maternal race/ethnicity and one-month exclusive breastfeeding in association with the in-hospital feeding modality. *Breastfeeding Medicine, 2*, 92-98.

Piper, S., & Parks, P. L. (2001). Use of an intensity ratio to describe breastfeeding exclusivity in a national sample. *Journal of Human Lactation, 17*, 227–232.

Preer, G.L., Newby, P.K., & Philipp, B.L. (2012). Weight loss in exclusively breastfed infants delivered by cesarean birth. *Journal of Human Lactation, 28*, 153-158.

Ratner, B. (1935). The treatment of milk allergy and its basic principles. *Journal of the American Medical Association, 105*, 934–939.

Reynolds, G.J., & Davies, S. (1993). A clinical audit of cotside blood glucose measurement in the detection of neonatal hypoglycemia. *Journal Pediatric Child Health, 29*, 289–291.

Rocha, N.M.N., Martinez, F.E., & Jorge, S.M. (2002). Cup or bottle for preterm infants: Effects on oxygen saturation, weight gain, and breastfeeding. *Journal of Human Lactation, 18*, 132–138.

Rodriguez ,G., Ventura, P., Samper, M.P., Moreno, L., Sarria, A., & Perez-Gonzalez, J.M. (2000). Changes in body composition during the initial hours of life in breastfed healthy term newborns. *Biology of the Neonate, 77*, 12–16.

Rosenberg, K.D., Eastham, C.A., Kasehagen, L.J., & Sandoval A.P. (2008). Marketing infant formula through hospitals: The impact of commercial hospital discharge packs on breastfeeding. *American Journal of Public Health, 98*, 290–295.

Rozance, P.J. (2013). Update on neonatal hypoglycemia. *Current Opinion Endocrinology Diabetes Obesity, 20,* [Ahead of print].

Rubaltelli, F.F. (1968). The frequency of neonatal hyperbilirubinemia in newborns with vacuum extractor. *Attualita di ostetricia e ginecologia, 14,* 1–4.

Ruth-Sanchez, V., & Greene, C.V. (1997). Water intoxication in a three day old: A case presentation. *Mother Baby Journal, 2,* 5–11.

Saarinen, K.M., Juntunen-Backman, K., Järvenpää, A.L., Klemetti, P., Kuitunen, P., Lope, L., ... Savilahti, E. (2000). Breast-feeding and the development of cows' milk protein allergy. *Advances in Experimental Medicine and Biology, 478,* 121-30.

Sakashita, R., Kamegai, T., & Inoue, N. (1996). Masseter muscle activity in bottle feeding with the chewing type bottle teat: Evidence from electromyographs. *Early Human Development, 45,* 83–92.

Salas, A.A., Salazar, J., Burgoa, C.V., De-Villegas, C.A., Quevedo, V., & Soliz, A. (2009). Significant weight loss in breastfed term infants readmitted for hyperbilirubinemia. *BMC Pediatrics, 9,* 82.

Santoro, W., Martinez, F.E., Ricco, R.G., & Jorge, S.M. (2010). Colostrum ingested during the first day of life by exclusively breastfed healthy newborn infants. *Journal of Pediatrics, 156,* 29-32.

Sarasua, I., Clausen, C., & Frunchak, V. (2009). Mothers' experiences with breastfeeding management and support: A quality improvement study. *Breastfeeding Review, 17,* 19-27.

Sase, M., Miwa, I., Sumie, M., Nakata, M., Suqino, N., Okada, K., ... Ross, M.G. (2005). Gastric emptying cycles in the human fetus. *American Journal of Obstetrics and Gynecology, 193,* 1000–1004.

Sato, H., Uchida, T., Toyota, K., Kanno, M., Hasimoto, T., Watanabe, M., ...Hayasaka, K. (2013). Association of breast-fed neonatal hyperbilirubinemia with UGT1A1 polymorphism: 211G>A (G71R) mutation becomes a risk factor under inadequate feeding. *Journal of Human Genetics, 58,* 7-10.

Scammon, R.E., & Doyle, L.O. (1920). Observations on the capacity of the stomach in the first ten days of postnatal life. *American Journal of Diseases of Children, 20,* 516–538.

Scariati, P.D., Grummer-Strawn, L.M., & Fein, S.B. (1997). Water supplementation of infants in the first month of life. *Archives of Pediatric Adolescent Medicine, 151,* 830–832.

Segami, Y., Mizuno, M., Taki, M., & Itabashi, K. (2013). Perioral movements and sucking pattern during bottle feeding with a novel, experimental teat are similar to breastfeeding. *Journal of Perinatology, 33,* 319-323.

Semenic, S., Loiselle, C., & Gottlieb, L. (2008). Predictors of the duration of exclusive breastfeeding among first-time mothers. *Research in Nursing & Health, 31,* 428-441.

Shrago, L. (1987). Glucose water supplementation of the breastfed infant during the first three days of life. *Journal of Human Lactation, 3,* 82–86.

Shrago, L.C., Reifsnider, E., & Insel, K. (2006).The Neonatal Bowel Output Study: Indicators of adequate breast milk intake in neonates. *Pediatric Nursing, 32,* 195-201.

Sievers, E., Haase, S., Oldigs, H.D., & Schaub, J. (2003). The impact of peripartum factors on the onset and duration of lactation. *Biology of the Neonate, 83,* 246-252.

Singh, G., Chouhan, R., & Sidhu, K. (2009). Effect of antenatal expression of breast milk at term in reducing breastfeeding failures. *Medical Journal Armed Forces India, 65,* 131-133.

Spangler, A.K., Randenberg, A.L., Brenner, M.G., & Howett, M. (2008). Belly models as teaching tools: What is their utility? *Journal of Human Lactation, 24*, 199–205.

Srinivasan, G., Pildes, R.S., Cattamanchi, G., Voora, S., & Lilien, L.D. (1986). Plasma glucose values in normal neonates: A new look. *Journal of Pediatrics, 109*, 114–117.

Stellwagen, L.M., Hubbard, E.T., & Wolf, A. (2007). The late preterm infant: A little baby with big needs. *Contemporary Pediatrics, 4*, 51-59.

Stettler, N., Stallings, V.A., Troxel, A.B., Zhao, J., Schinnar, R., Nelson, S.E., ... Strom, B.L. (2005). Weight gain in the first week of life and overweight in adulthood: A cohort study of European American subjects fed infant formula. *Circulation, 111*, 1897-1903.

Stewart, J.A., Chadwick, V.S., & Murray, A. (2006). Carriage, quantification, and predominance of methanogens and sulfate-reducing bacteria in fecal samples. *Letters in Applied Microbiology, 43,* 58–63.

Stratton, J.F., Stronge, J., & Boylan, P.C. (1995). Hyponatremia and non-electrolyte solutions in labouring primigravida. *European Journal Obstetrics Gynaecology Reproductive Biology, 59*, 149–151.

Swenne, I., Ewald, U., Gustafsson, J., Sandberg, E., & Ostenson, C.G. (1994). Inter-relationship between serum concentrations of glucose, glucagon, and insulin during the first two days of life in healthy newborns. *Acta Pediatrica, 83*, 915–919.

Taveras, E.M., Li, R., Grummer-Strawn, L., Richardson, M., Marshall, R., Rego, V.H., Miroshnik, I., & Lieu, T.A. (2004). Opinions and practices of clinicians associated with continuation of exclusive breastfeeding. *Pediatrics, 113*, e283-e290.

Taylor, S.N., Basile, L.A., Ebeling, M., & Wagner, C.L. (2009). Intestinal permeability in preterm infants by feeding type: Mother's milk versus formula. *Breastfeeding Medicine, 4,* 11-15.

Tender, J.A.F., Janakiram, J., Arce, E., Mason, R., Jordan, T., Marsh, J., ... Moon, R.Y. (2009). Reasons for in-hospital formula supplementation of breastfed infants from low-income families. *Journal of Human Lactation, 25,* 11–17.

Tornese, G., Ronfani, L., Pavan, C., Demarini, S., Monasta, L., & Davavzo, R. (2012). Does the LATCH score assessed in the first 24 hours after delivery predict non-exclusive breastfeeding at hospital discharge? *Breastfeeding Medicine, 7*, 423-430.

Tozier, P.K. (2013). Colostrum versus formula supplementation for glucose stabilization in newborns of diabetic mothers. *Journal of Obstetric, Gynecologic, and Neonatal Nursing, 42*, 619-628.

Unal, S., Arhan, E., Kara, N., Uncu, N., & Alliefendioglu, D. (2008). Breastfeeding-associated hypernatremia: Retrospective analysis of 169 term newborns. *Pediatrics International, 50*, 29–34.

United States Lactation Consultant Association. (2010). *International board certified lactation consultant staffing recommendations for the inpatient setting.* Morrisville, NC. http://uslca.org/wp-content/uploads/2013/02/IBCLC_Staffing_Recommendations_July_2010.pdf

Uras, N., Karadag, A., Dogan, G., Tonbul, A., & Tatli, M.M. (2007). Moderate hypernatremic dehydration in newborn infants: Retrospective evaluation of 64 cases. *Journal Maternal Fetal Neonatal Medicine, 20*, 449–452.

Van den Driessche, M., Peeters, K., Marien, P., Ghoos, Y., Devileger, H., & Veerman-Wauters, G. (1999). Gastric emptying in formula-fed and breastfed infants measured with the 13C-octanoic acid breath test. *Journal of Pediatric Gastroenterology Nutrition, 29*, 46–51.

Verhasselt, V. (2010). Neonatal tolerance under breastfeeding influence. *Current Opinion in Immunology, 22,* 5, 623-630.

Waldrop, J. (2013). Exploration of reasons for feeding choices in Hispanic mothers. *MCN American Journal of Maternal and Child Nursing, 38,* 282-288.

Walker, M. (2007). *Still selling out mothers and babies: Marketing of breastmilk substitutes in the USA.* Weston, MA: National Alliance for Breastfeeding Advocacy.

Walters, M.W., Boggs, K.M., Ludington-Hoe, S., Price, K.M., & Morrison, B. (2007). Kangaroo care at birth for full term infants: A pilot study. *American Journal of Maternal Child Nursing, 32,* 375–381.

Watson, J., Hodnett, E., Armson, A., Davies, B., & Watt-Watson, J. (2012). A randomized controlled trial of the effect of intrapartum intravenous fluid management on breastfed newborn weight loss. *Journal of Obstetric Gynecologic Neonatal Nursing, 41,* 24-32.

Werner, E.F., Janevic, T.M., Illuzzi, J., Funai, E.F., Savitz, D.A., & Lipkind, H.S. (2011). Mode of delivery in nulliparous women and neonatal intracranial injury. *Obstetrics & Gynecology, 118,* 1239-1246.

Widstrom, A.M., Christensson, K., Ransjo-Arvidson, A.B., Matthiesen, A.S., Winberg, J., & Uvnas-Moberg, K. (1988). Gastric aspirates of newborn infants: pH, volume and levels of gastrin- and somatostatin-like immunoreactivity. *Acta Paediatrica Scandinavia, 77,* 502–508.

Wight, N.E. (2001). *Supplements and the breastfed infant: When are they needed and how should they be supplied?* Independent Study Module. Schaumburg, IL: La Leche League International.

Wight, N.E. (2006). Hypoglycemia in breastfed neonates. *Breastfeeding Medicine, 1,* 253–262.

Wight, N., Marinelli, K.A., Academy of Breastfeeding Medicine Protocol Committee. (2006). ABM clinical protocol #1: Guidelines for glucose monitoring and treatment of hypoglycemia in breastfed neonates. Revision June, 2006. *Breastfeeding Medicine, 3,* 178-184.

Williams, A.F. (1997). *Hypoglycemia of the newborn: Review of the literature.* Geneva: World Health Organization.

Winberg, J. (2005). Mother and newborn baby: Mutual regulation of physiology and behavior-a selective review. *Developmental Psychobiology, 47,* 217-229.

Wojcicki, J.M., Holbrook, K., Lustig, R.H., Caughey, A.B., Munoz, R.F., Heyman, M.B. (2011). Infant formula, tea, and water supplementation of Latino infants at 4-6 weeks postpartum. *Journal of Human Lactation, 27,* 122-130.

Wolf, J.H. (2001). *Don't kill your baby: Public health and the decline of breastfeeding in the nineteenth and twentieth centuries.* Columbus, OH: The Ohio State University Press.

Wolf, L.S., & Glass, R.P. (1992). *Feeding and swallowing disorders in infancy.* Tucson, AZ: Therapy Skill Builders.

World Health Organization. (2009). *Acceptable medical reasons for use of breast-milk substitutes.* Geneva, Switzerland. http://whqlibdoc.who.int/hq/2009/WHO_FCH_CAH_09.01_eng.pdf

Yamauchi, Y., & Yamanouchi, I. (1990). Breastfeeding frequency during the first 24 hours after birth in full term neonates. *Pediatrics, 86,* 171–175.

Yang, W.C, Zhao, L.L., Li, Y.C., Chen, C.H., Chang, Y.J., Fu, Y.C., & Wu, H.P. (2013). Bodyweight loss in predicting neonatal hyperbilirubinemia 72 hours after birth in term newborn infants. *BMC Pediatrics, 13,* 145.

Yilmaz, G., Caylan, N., Karacan, C.D., Bodur, I., & Gokcay, G. (2014). Effect of cup feeding and bottle feeding on breastfeeding in late preterm infants: A randomized controlled study. *Journal of Human Lactation*, Ahead of print. DOI: 10.1177/0890334413517940.

Zangen, S., Di Lorenzo, C., Zangen, T., Mertz, H., Schwankovsky, L., & Hyman, P.E. (2001). Rapid maturation of gastric relaxation in newborn infants. *Pediatric Research, 50*, 629–632.

Zhang, A.Q., Lee, S.Y.R., Truneh, M., Everett, M.L., & Parker, W. (2012). Human whey promotes sessile bacterial growth, whereas alternative sources of infant nutrition promote planktonic growth. *Current Nutrition & Food Science, 8*, 168-176.

Index

About The Author

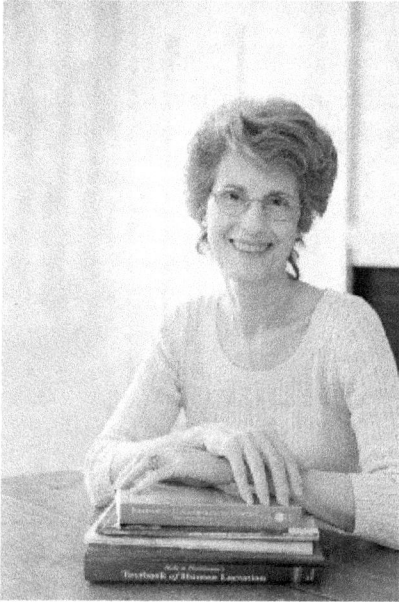

Marsha Walker, RN, IBCLC is the Executive Director of the National Alliance for Breastfeeding Advocacy, Research, Education and Legal Branch (NABA REAL). She is a long-time breastfeeding advocate, starting as a volunteer breastfeeding counselor with the Nursing Mothers Counsel in California. Marsha went on to become a childbirth educator through Lamaze International, a registered nurse, and an International Board Certified Lactation Consultant. She served on the Representative Panel of Experts in 1985, which constructed the first lactation consultant exam and was one of a number of clinicians on whose practice the exam grid is based. Marsha enjoyed a large clinical lactation practice at Harvard Pilgrim Health Plan, a major HMO in Massachusetts, where she was the Director of the Breastfeeding Support Program for 12 years. She has served on the Board of Directors of the International Lactation Consultant Association (ILCA) for seven years, including as its president in 1999.

Marsha is on the Board of Directors of the Massachusetts Breastfeeding Coalition, Baby Friendly USA, the US Lactation Consultant Association, and Best for Babes. She is the US Lactation Consultant Association's representative to the U.S. Department of Agriculture's Breastfeeding Promotion Consortium and NABA's representative to the U.S. Breastfeeding Committee. She worked for eight years to get breastfeeding legislation passed in her state of Massachusetts, which became a reality in January 2009. She is the chair of the Ban the Bags campaign, a national effort to eliminate the hospital distribution of formula company discharge bags.

NABA REAL is the IBFAN organization in the United States and is responsible for monitoring the International Code of Marketing of Breastmilk Substitutes in the U.S. Marsha has written both country reports on Code monitoring activities in the U.S., "Selling Out Mothers and Babies" and "Still Selling Out Mothers and Babies." Marsha is an international speaker on breastfeeding and an author of numerous publications, including her book *Breastfeeding Management for the Clinician: Using the Evidence.*

Marsha is married and the mother of two breastfed children, Shannon and Justin, her original breastfeeding clinical instructors. She is the grandmother of five breastfed children - Haley, Sophie, Isabelle, Ella, and Andrew.

Note from the Author

Dear Reader,

Thank you for purchasing and reading this book. I hope you enjoyed it. If it was helpful to you, you can help me reach other readers by writing a review of the book on Amazon.com and/or ibreastfeeding.com.

Sincerely,

Marsha Walker